全国高等学校教材

供临床、预防、基础、口腔、药学、护理等专业用

教师用书

医学专业英语

阅读一分册

总主编　白永权

主　编　范晓晖

副主编　李永安　熊淋宵

编　委　（按姓氏笔画排序）

王　丹　陕西中医药大学

白永权　西安交通大学

朱　元　西安交通大学

李永安　陕西中医药大学

李权芳　陕西中医药大学

张　鹏　西安交通大学

范晓晖　西安交通大学

易　超　西安交通大学

晏国莉　西安交通大学

熊淋宵　北京中医药大学

穆文超　陕西中医药大学

人民卫生出版社

·北　京·

图书在版编目(CIP)数据

医学专业英语. 阅读一分册教师用书 / 范晓晖主编
. —北京：人民卫生出版社，2021.12
ISBN 978-7-117-32454-0

Ⅰ. ①医… Ⅱ. ①范… Ⅲ. ①医学－英语－阅读教学－医学院校－教学参考资料 Ⅳ. ①R

中国版本图书馆 CIP 数据核字（2021）第 235570 号

医学专业英语 阅读一分册教师用书
Yixue Zhuanye Yingyu Yuedu Yi Fence Jiaoshi Yongshu

主　　编：范晓晖
出版发行：人民卫生出版社（中继线 010-59780011）
地　　址：北京市朝阳区潘家园南里 19 号
邮　　编：100021
E - mail：pmph @ pmph.com
购书热线：010-59787592　010-59787584　010-65264830
印　　刷：河北新华第一印刷有限责任公司
经　　销：新华书店
开　　本：787 × 1092　1/16　　印张：5
字　　数：122 千字
版　　次：2021 年 12 月第 1 版
印　　次：2021 年 12 月第 1 次印刷
标准书号：ISBN 978-7-117-32454-0
定　　价：30.00 元

修订说明

《医学专业英语》系列教材自2001年出版以来，深受广大医学英语教师、医学生和医务工作者的欢迎，许多医学院校一直在使用，先后印刷二十多次。我国香港特别行政区和国外一些医学院校也以不同的方式选用了该套教材。2016年人民卫生出版社决定对这套教材进行修订，我们再次组织全国医学院校中精通医学英语教学和教材编写的老师，包括部分参加过编写第1版教材的老师，在保留原有教材实用、专业和规范的特点和风格同时，对该套教材进行了一次认真、全面的修改，使之更贴近医学生的学习需求，更好地满足我国医学英语教学的需要，进一步体现教材服务于医学教育和追踪医学科学发展前沿的本质，切实提高医学生的医学英语应用能力。

本次修订的重点是对全套教材进行重新梳理，改正第1版教材中的疏漏之处；适当降低全套教材的难度；适度压缩各分册的内容；调整某些章节的先后顺序；删除教学效果不佳和不符合当前教学实际要求的课文和练习；换入一批可读性更强、体现医学科学最新知识的文章和更能培养学生英语语言输出能力的练习。

本次修订的原则如下。

1. 本套教材的修订以《大学英语教学指南》为指导，依据当代专门用途英语教学理念，引用网络和多媒体等现代教育技术，进行修订和编写。本套教材的原有定位不变，以我国大学英语四级水平为起点，供临床、预防、基础、口腔、药学和护理等专业的本科生和硕士研究生学习使用。

2. 修订后本套教材共六册，其中学生用书三册：《医学专业英语　阅读一分册》《医学专业英语　阅读二分册》（合称《阅读分册》）和《医学专业英语　听说分册》（简称《听说分册》）；教师用书三册：《医学专业英语　阅读一分册教师用书》《医学专业英语　阅读二分册教师用书》和《医学专业英语　听说分册教师用书》。

3. 阅读、听说两种教材都独立自成体系，但又相互关联形成一个整体。在教学中每种教材既可单独使用，也可根据实际需要将两种教材组合在一起使用。每册教材可满足40学时的课内教学使用，全套教材可供120学时的教学使用。

4.《阅读分册》与《听说分册》每章的主题基本相同，都是同一个医学人体系统。在编写英语系列教材时，采用每册中每章主题相同的编写模式既是对英语教材编写体例的创新，也更适合医学英语教学。学生从阅读和听说不同角度学习同一个医学人体系统的常用医学英语术语构词形式和该系统人体结构、生理和常见疾病的英语词汇和英语表述。

医学英语是很多国家和地区的医学生都要学习的一门课程，差异只是学时的多少和内容的深浅。母语是英语的医学生只学习医学英语词汇学，而母语是非英语的医学生需要将普通英语和医学英语结合起来，起点低而且学时多。在本套教材的修订和编写过程中，我们充分考虑到了我国医学英语教育的现状以及医学生学习医学英语的实际需要和存在的难点，力争编写出一套适合我国医学英语教学的优秀医学英语教材。

本次修订中，各位编者认真负责，对每个分册都进行了大幅度的调整和改编。新版《听说分册》增加了大量新音频，使得语料更加真实活泼；《阅读分册》新选了许多可读性更强的文章，同时对原书每篇文章的长度都做了适当压缩。在练习的配置方面，更加突出了对医学生英语语言输出能力的培养，增加了大量说、写和译的练习。

《医学专业英语》系列教材第 1 版和第 2 版都由白永权教授担任总主编。第 1 版的《医学专业英语　阅读一分册》由邱望生担任主编，郝长江担任副主编，编者有陈忠荣、张帆和郝军；《医学专业英语　阅读二分册》由张宏清担任主编，周铁成担任副主编，编者有胡建、葛广纯、王群英和孙秋丹；《医学专业英语　听说分册》由董双辰担任主编，梁平担任副主编，编者有王文秀、陈春林和潘宏声。第 2 版的《医学专业英语　阅读一分册》及教师用书由范晓晖担任主编，李永安、熊淋宵担任副主编，编者有朱元、王丹、李权芳、易超、穆文超、晏国莉和张鹏；《医学专业英语　阅读二分册》及教师用书由卢凤香担任主编，吴青担任副主编，编者有谢春晖、任雁、华瑶、杨波、王梦杰和郑艳华；《医学专业英语　听说分册》及教师用书由陈向京担任主编，孙庆祥担任副主编，编者有李莹、晏国莉、戴月珍、凌秋虹、詹菊红和陈英。

参加《医学专业英语》系列教材两版编写的院校有西安交通大学、北京大学、复旦大学、首都医科大学、北京中医药大学、青岛大学、陕西中医药大学、四川大学、华中科技大学、中南大学、吉林大学、中山大学、南方医科大学、海军军医大学（原第二军医大学）、陆军军医大学（原第三军医大学）、空军军医大学（原第四军医大学）、哈尔滨医科大学、河北医科大学、山东大学、兰州大学和承德医学院。

本次修订过程中，许多教授、学者和领导付出了很大心血，在此对他们表示衷心的感谢。

《医学专业英语》系列教材出版以来，我们收集到了一些宝贵意见和建议，这为我们做好第 2 版的修订工作提供了十分宝贵和可靠的依据和资料。在此谨向提出意见和建议的各位读者，向所有使用这套教材的老师和同学，表示深深的敬意和感谢，欢迎你们今后一如既往地不吝指教。

白永权

2021 年 8 月

前　言

本书为《医学专业英语》系列教材的阅读第一分册的教师用书，以我国大学英语四级水平为起点，供临床、预防、基础、口腔、药学和护理等专业的本科生和硕士研究生学习医学专业英语使用。

编写宗旨

《医学专业英语　阅读一分册》旨在帮助学生学习人体解剖系统的英语术语以及人体各系统结构、生理和常见疾病的英语词汇和英语表达，通过听、说、读、写、译多方面进行医学英语语言知识的操练，培养学生的医学英语语言表达能力和综合应用能力。

全书框架

本册共 9 章，分别为人体概论、疾病概论、肌肉系统、骨骼系统、消化系统、呼吸系统、心血管系统、血液和免疫以及发育和遗传。每章都包括医学词汇（Medical Terminology）和阅读短文（Reading Passages）两大部分。

Section A　Medical Terminology

医学词汇部分每章都讲授 20 个左右本系统常用的构词形式和前后缀，并配有 3 类有利于医学词汇学习和记忆的练习。

Section B　Reading Passages

阅读部分每章都包括 3 篇有关人体同一系统或同一主题的文章，除了第一、二和九章外，每章的主题是一个人体解剖系统，学生将学习该系统的常用医学英语术语构词形式和该系统人体结构、生理功能和常见疾病的英语词汇和英语表达。第 1 篇是关于该系统解剖和生理功能的短文；第 2 篇是有关该系统病理和疾病的概述；第 3 篇是该系统的某个特定疾病。3 篇文章的内容由浅入深、相互呼应，难度和长度逐篇加大。

第 1 篇和第 2 篇文章后各配 4 个大练习。每个练习都有明确的目的。

- 配对和句子填空类练习考查学生对本课基本词汇和主要知识的掌握。
- 段落填空类练习进一步训练学生的语句表达技能，强调语句内在的逻辑关系和语义关联。
- 短语、句子和段落的汉英及英汉翻译类练习培养学生的语言综合应用能力。
- 任务型口头回答问题类练习培养学生学以致用的口语表达能力。

第 3 篇文章后配有两类大练习。

- 判断正误或多项选择类练习考查学生对课文主旨大意和重要细节的理解。
- 医学词汇构成分析类练习进一步培养学生运用构词法知识辨识单词意思的能力。

为了便于读者学习和查阅生词，在本书的后面附有总词汇表。

本册阅读可供40学时的教学使用。在具体使用时，根据学生的英语水平和课程时数决定是全部使用，还是选用某一部分或某几篇文章。一般来说，词汇部分是必学的，阅读部分的3篇文章可根据学生的不同水平来选用，剩余的文章留给学有余力的学生自学。

修订特色

结合我国医学英语教育的现状以及医学生学习医学英语的实际需要，在保持第一版原有定位和特色的前提下，本册教材修订的总体目标是使本教材更贴近医学英语教学的实际需要和学生的实际水平。修订的重点是适当降低难度和更换教学效果不佳或不太符合当前教学实际的课文和练习。为此，我们对本书主要做了以下两方面的修订：

- 更换了原书近三分之一的文章，删除了原书中内容过时或过于专业、语言难度过大的文章，新选了一批可读性更强、更具时代感的文章。
- 对所有练习的形式和内容进行了必要的修改，对原有的练习重新排序，使其更符合由易到难循序渐进的学习原则。

本书由范晓晖担任分册主编，李永安、熊淋宵担任分册副主编，朱元、王丹、李权芳、易超、穆文超、晏国莉和张鹏参与编写。

由于时间紧迫和编者水平有限，书中难免会存在缺点和错误，望同行和读者不吝赐教。

编　者

2021年8月

Contents

Chapter One Human Body as a Whole

Section A Medical Terminology

Learn the following combining forms, prefixes and suffixes and write the meanings of the medical terms in the space provided.

Word Part	Meaning	Example Term	Meaning in English and Chinese
a-, an- (in front of vowel)	not, without 无	asexual /eɪ'sekʃʊəl/	not having or involving sex 无性的
		acentric /eɪ'sentrɪk/	not centered, having no center 无中心的
		anoxia /æ'nɒksɪə/ (*ox/i* oxygen)	without oxygen 缺氧，无氧
		anuria /ə'njʊərɪə/ (*ur/o* urine)	without urine 无尿
aden/o	gland 腺体	adenvirus /'ædɪnəʊˌvaɪrəs/	any of a group of viruses that cause respiratory infections 腺病毒
		adenomegaly /ˌədɪnəʊ'megəlɪ/ (*-megaly* enlargement)	enlargement of the gland 腺体肥大
-al	pertaining to ……的	renal /'riːnəl/ (*ren/o* kidney)	pertaining to the kidney 肾脏的，肾的
		nasal /'neɪzəl/ (*nas/o* nose)	pertaining to the nose 鼻的
-algia	pain 疼痛	analgia /ə'nældʒɪə/	without pain, lack of pain 无痛觉
		neuralgia /njʊə'rældʒɪə/	pain of the nerves 神经痛
-ar	pertaining to ……的	vascular /'væskjʊlə/ (*vascul/o* blood vessel)	pertaining to blood vessels 血管的
		cellular /'seljʊlə/	pertaining to the cell 细胞的
auto-	self 自己的；自动的	autograft /'ɔːtəʊgrɑːft/	a transplant tissue obtained from the patient's own body 自体移植
		autonomous /ɔː'tɔːnəməs/	able to govern itself or control its own affairs 自制的，自律的
bi/o	life 生物，生命	biosphere /'baɪəʊsfɪə/	regions of the atmosphere of the earth where living organisms exist 生物圈
		biology /baɪ'ɒlədʒɪ/ (*-logy* the study of)	study of life 生物学
cardi/o	heart 心脏	cardiomegaly /ˌkɑːdɪəʊ'megəlɪ/	enlargement of the heart 心脏肥大
		cardiology /ˌkɑːdɪ'ɒlədʒɪ/	study of the heart 心脏病学；心脏学

Continue

Word Part	Meaning	Example Term	Meaning in English and Chinese
-cele	hernia 疝 protrusion 膨出	cardiocele /'kaːdɪəʊsiːl/	protrusion of the heart 心膨出
		adenocele /'ədɪnəʊsiːl/	protrusion of the gland 腺膨出，腺囊肿
chrom/o, chromat/o	color 色彩，颜色	chromosome /'krəʊməsəʊm/ (*-some* body)	the color body, the substance in the cell that carries genetic features 染色体
		achromia /ə'krəʊmɪə/	without color, colorless 无色的
		chromatology /ˌkrəʊmə'tɒlədʒɪ/	study of color 色彩学
		chromatic /krə'mætɪk/	pertaining to color 色的
cyt/o	cell 细胞	cytolysis /saɪ'tɒləsɪs/ (*-lysis* breaking down)	breaking down of the cell 细胞溶解
		cytology /saɪ'tɒlədʒɪ/	study of the cell 细胞学
encephal/o	brain 脑	encephalopathy /ˌensefə'lɔpəθɪ/ (*-pathy* disease)	disease of the brain 脑病
		encephalocele /en'sefələʊsiːl/	hernia or protrusion of the brain 脑疝
-ectomy	excision 切除	gastrectomy /gæs'trektəmɪ/ (*gastr/o* stomach)	excision of the stomach 胃切除术
		adenectomy /ˌædə'nektəmɪ/	excision of the gland 腺切除术
endo-	inner 内	endocrinology /ˌendəʊkrɪ'nɒlədʒɪ/	study of the endocrine system 内分泌学
		endocardial /ˌendəʊ'kaːdɪəl/	pertaining to the inner lining of the heart or inside the heart 心内的；心内膜的
ex-	out 外；出	exhale /eks'heɪl/	breathe out 呼气
		expel /ɪk'spel/ (*pel/* drive)	drive out 驱逐
-gen	origin 原 producer 产生物	pathogen /'pæθədʒən/	disease-producing agent 病原体
		carcinogen /kaː'sɪnədʒən/ (*carcin/o* cancer)	cancer-producing agent 致癌物
hepat/o	liver 肝	hepatitis /ˌhepə'taɪtɪs/	inflammation of the liver 肝炎
		hepatectomy /ˌhepə'tektəmɪ/	excision of the liver 肝切除术
hist/o	tissue 组织	histology /hɪ'stɒlədʒɪ/	study of the tissue 组织学
		histolysis /hɪ'stɒlɪsɪs/	breaking down of the tissue 组织溶解
-ic	pertaining to 关于 relating to ……的	thoracic /θɔː'ræsɪk/ (*thorac/o* chest)	pertaining to the chest 胸部的，胸腔的
		toxic /'tɒksɪk/	relating to or caused by a toxin 有毒的
-itis	inflammation 炎症	arthritis /ɑː'θraɪtɪs/ (arthr/o joint)	inflammation of the joint 关节炎
		adenitis /ˌædə'naɪtɪs/	inflammation of the gland 腺炎
-logy	the study of ……学	neurology /njʊ'rɔːlədʒɪ/	study of the nerve 神经学
		hepatology /ˌhepə'tɒlədʒɪ/	study of the liver and its diseases 肝脏病学
-plasm	formation 形成物 substance 浆；质	cytoplasm /'saɪtəʊˌplæzəm/	jelly substance in the cell 胞质
		neoplasm /'niːəʊˌplæzəm/ (neo- new)	new formation, new growth 新生物，肿瘤
-tomy	incision 切开术 process of cutting 切断术	encephalotomy /ˌensefə'ləʊtəʊmɪ/	incision into the brain 脑切开术
		cardiotomy /ˌkaːdɪ'ɒtəmɪ/	incision into the heart 心脏切开术

Exercises

Ⅰ. Complete each of the following sentences with a correct word part.

1. Word beginnings are called prefixes.
2. Word endings are called suffixes.
3. The foundation of a word is known as the root.
4. A vowel linking two roots or linking a root with a suffix in a term is called a combining vowel.
5. The combination of a root and a combining vowel is known as the combining form.

Ⅱ. Add suffix -logy to the following combining forms and explain their meanings. The first one has been provided for you.

Combining forms	Term	Meaning
1. cardi/o	cardiology	study of the heart
2. hepat/o	hepatology	study of the liver
3. aden/o	adenology	study of the gland
4. bi/o	biology	study of life
5. cyt/o	cytology	study of the cell
6. encephal/o	encephalology	study of the brain
7. hist/o	histology	study of the tissue
8. chromat/o	chromatology	study of color

Ⅲ. Match each word part in Column A with its English term in Column B. Write the corresponding letter in the blank provided.

	Column A(Word Parts)	Column B(English Terms)
E	1. a-, an-	A. hernia, protrusion
G	2. chrom/o	B. pain
A	3. -cele	C. life
B	4. -algia	D. formation, substance of formation
M	5. cyt/o	E. not, without
D	6. -plasm	F. inner, within
F	7. endo-	G. color
N	8. cardi/o	H. gland
H	9. aden/o	I. tissue
I	10. hist/o	J. brain
O	11. hepat/o	K. incision
J	12. encephal/o	L. self
L	13. auto-	M. cell
K	14. -tomy	N. heart
C	15. bi/o	O. liver

Section B Reading Passages

Passage One The Human Body

Exercises

Ⅰ. Match each term in Column A with its corresponding description in Column B. Write the corresponding letter in the blank provided.

	Column A	Column B
F	1. cytology	A. a liquid produced by the liver which helps to digest fat
B	2. metabolism	B. the physical and chemical processes by which living substance is maintained and energy is produced
I	3. cartilage	C. nourishing substance
G	4. lymph	D. any of the minute blood vessels connecting arterioles with venules
H	5. trachea	E. chemical substance produced by various endocrine glands
D	6. capillary	F. the branch of biology that studies the structure and function of cells
A	7. bile	G. colorless fluid from the tissues or organs of the body, containing white blood cells
J	8. hematology	H. a membranous tube that conveys inhaled air from the larynx to the bronchi
C	9. nutrient	I. a strong, flexible substance in the body, especially around the joints
E	10. hormone	J. the study of blood

Ⅱ. Fill in each blank with one proper word.

Several fields are involved in the study of the human body. (1) Anatomy focuses on the structure and form of the human body. Human (2) physiology studies the functioning of the human body, including its systems, tissues, and cells. The study of tissues is the focus of (3) histology, and the study of cells is part of (4) cytology. The human body's cells, tissues, organs, and systems work together in remarkable harmony. Actions as simple as eating a piece of fruit involve numerous (5) systems in complex coordination, whether the (6) nervous system, with impulses traveling up to 248 mph, or the (7) muscular system, with contracting and relaxation of some of the body's 600 muscles, or the (8) endocrine system, involving hormones produced by glands in one part of the body that affect selecting cells with the correct receptors in (9) other parts of the body. Should one organ or system of the body fail in performing its (10) function, the entire body is affected.

Ⅲ. Translate the following into English.

1. 心血管疾病	cardiovascular disease	2. 分子	molecule
3. 泌尿道	urethra	4. 内分泌学	endocrinology

5. 动脉	artery	6. 神经系统	nervous system
7. 组织学	histology	8. 血液循环	blood circulation
9. 免疫学	immunology	10.生理学	physiology
11.解剖学	anatomy	12.甲状腺	thyroid
13.胚胎学	embryology	14.生殖系统	reproductive system
15.新陈代谢	metabolism	16.脊髓	spinal cord

Ⅳ.Discuss the following topics.

1. Why do we study anatomy and physiology?

   We study anatomy and physiology to understand the human body. Anatomy studies how the body parts are put together while physiology studies how they function.

2. Suppose you were a professor of anatomy trying to introduce the human body to your students at the first class, where would you like to begin and how would you like to proceed?

   The answer is open.

3. Give a brief account of the structure and functions of each organ system.

   The skeletal system is made up of the bones, joints, and cartilage. Its functions are to provide support and protection for the soft tissues and the organs of the body and to provide points of attachment for the muscles.

   The muscular system consists of cardiac muscles, smooth muscles and skeletal muscles. Its functions are to allow the body to move, and its contractions produce heat, which helps maintain a constant body temperature.

   The circulatory system is made up of the heart, blood vessels, and the blood. Its functions are to distribute needed materials and remove unneeded ones.

   The respiratory system is made up of the mouth, nose, larynx, trachea, and lungs. It takes in oxygen form the air and expels carbon dioxide and water vapor.

   The digestive system consists of a tube extending from the mouth to the anus. Its functions are to break down the food and fluids into small molecules, and absorb them into the circulatory system.

   The urinary system involves the kidneys, ureters, bladder and urethra. Its function is to maintain normal levels of water and of certain small molecules such as sodium and potassium in the body.

   The endocrine system consists of many glands, such as the pituitary, thyroid, sex organs, adrenal gland, and pancreas. Its main function is to control body activities by means of hormones.

   The nervous system contains the brain, spinal cord and nerves. It also controls body activities.

   The reproductive system is constructed differently for males and females. Its functions are to manufacture cells that allow reproduction and produce sex hormones.

   The skin is a complete layer that protects the inner structures of the body. It keeps out foreign substances and prevents excessive water evaporation.

Passage Two Cells and Tissues

Exercises

Ⅰ. Translate the following into English.

1. 细胞核 nucleus
2. 高尔基体 Golgi apparatus
3. 细胞中心粒 centriole
4. 溶酶体 lysosome
5. 细胞质 cytoplasm
6. 细胞膜 cell membrane
7. 线粒体 mitochondrion
8. 核糖体 ribosome

Ⅱ. Fill in each blank with a correct word in the box. Change the form of the words if necessary.

voluntary	molecule	hereditary	genetic	connective
cytoplasm	homeostasis	carbohydrate	epithelial	membrane

1. Homeostasis is the property of a system in which variables are regulated so that internal conditions remain stable and relatively constant.
2. Cell nuclei contain most of the cell's genetic material, organized as multiple long linear DNA molecules in complex with a large variety of proteins to form chromosomes.
3. Much of the chemical work is performed in the cytoplasm.
4. Bread, potatoes, pasta and rice are all high in carbohydrates.
5. The tendency to become obese is at least in part hereditary.
6. The cells of epithelial tissue pack tightly together and form continuous sheets that serve as linings in different parts of the body.
7. Some examples of connective tissues include the inner layers of skin, tendons, ligaments, cartilage, bone and fat tissue.
8. The cell membrane is primarily composed of a mix of proteins and lipids.
9. A molecule of water consists of two atoms of hydrogen and one atom of oxygen.
10. Striated muscle, whose fibers appear striped under a microscope, is responsible for voluntary movement.

Ⅲ. Translate the following sentences into Chinese.

1. The average cell in the human body—about ten microns in diameter—is a speck barely visible without the aid of a microscope.
   一般的人体细胞直径为10μm，是一个不借助显微镜就基本上看不见的小点。
2. For one-celled organisms this fluid is an external body of water—the ocean, a lake, or a stream. For many-celled plants and animals, however, the medium is part of the organism—in plants, the sap; in animals, the blood.
   对于单细胞生物而言，这种液体是细胞外面的水，即海洋、湖泊或小溪；但对于多细胞的动植物而言，这种媒介就是生物体的一部分——对于植物来讲是它的汁液，对于动物来讲是它的血液。

3. Located along the endoplasmic reticulum as well as elsewhere in the cytoplasm are numerous ribosomes. These tiny granules consist in part of ribonucleic acid (RNA).
   大量的核糖体沿着内质网和细胞质各处分布，这些微小的颗粒组成了核糖核酸的一部分。
4. Enclosed by a two-layered membrane, the nucleus contains a liquid called nucleoplasm as well as strands of deoxyribonucleic acid (DNA) covered with a coating of protein.
   细胞核被两层膜包围，中心是核质（浆）及表面覆盖着蛋白质的脱氧核糖核酸链。
5. Cardiac and smooth muscles can function without conscious control and are thus described as involuntary muscle.
   心肌和平滑肌可以不受意识的控制发挥作用，故称为不随意肌。

Ⅳ. Discuss the following topics.

1. What are the vital parts of a cell?
   The vital parts of a cell are the cell membrane, the cytoplasm, and the nucleus.
2. Give a brief account of the structures and functions of the cell membrane, cytoplasm and nucleus.
   The cell membrane is an extremely thin but tough band of protein and phospholipid molecules. Its functions are to admit useful substances and to reject harmful substances from the surrounding fluid as well as to force out or excrete waste products into the fluid.
   The cytoplasm is mainly water. Its water content varies from a minimum of about 65 per cent to a maximum of about 95 per cent. The solids in the cytoplasm include granular proteins, carbohydrates, droplets of fat, and pigments. Most of the cell's constant work of keeping alive is performed in the cytoplasm.
   The nucleus is roundish or oval near the center of the cell. It is made up of a two-layered membrane, nucleoplasm, and strands of DNA. The nucleus controls the growth and division of the cell. It also contains the structures that transmit hereditary traits.
3. List the four types of tissues and briefly introduce their functions.
   The epithelial tissue covers and protects body structures and lines organs, vessels, and cavities. The connective tissue supports and binds body structures. The muscle tissue contracts to produce movement. The nervous tissue makes up the brain, spinal cord, and nerves. It coordinates and controls body responses by transmitting electrical impulses.

Passage Three The Practice of Medicine

Exercises

Ⅰ. Read the following statements and decide whether they are true or false. Then write T for true and F for false in the brackets.

1. [T] The rapid development of science and technology in the twenty-first century has changed the way doctors practice medicine.
2. [F] When taking a patient's history, the doctor just needs to list all the reported or observed symptoms.

3. [T] The family history can indicate the likelihood of certain diseases, such as coronary heart disease and high blood pressure.
4. [T] Doctors should record the results of physical examination in time to prevent inaccuracy.
5. [F] Physical examination should not be repeated too often in order to minimize the patient's suffering.
6. [F] With the development of various laboratory tests, physicians no longer need to spend too much time examining the patient.
7. [F] Genomics studies the changes in chromatin and histone proteins and methylation of DNA sequences that affect gene expression.
8. [T] Proteomics, microbiomics and metagenomics, which study genetic and environmental factors affecting health, are making rapid progress.

Ⅱ. Here is a list of terms from the text. Analyze their meanings using the word building knowledge you have learned. Leave the space empty if the word part does not apply.

Term	Prefix	Combining Form/Root	Suffix	Chinese Translation
1. pathophysiology		path/o physi/o	-logy	病理生理学
2. hyperthyroidism	hyper-	thyr/o	-oid -ism	甲状腺功能亢进
3. genotyping		gen(e) type	-ing	基因分型
4. pandemic	pan-	dem	-ic	大流行的
5. phenotype	pheno-	type		表现型
6. microbiomics	micro-	bio	-omics	微生物组学

Chapter Two Diseases and Disorders

Section A Medical Terminology

Learn the following combining forms, prefixes and suffixes and write the meanings of the medical terms in the space provided.

Word Part	Meaning	Example Term	Meaning in English and Chinese
adip/o	fat 脂肪	adiposis /ˌædɪ'pəʊsɪs/ (*-osis* abnormal condition)	excessive fatness 脂肪过多症
		adipocyte /'ædɪpəʊˌsaɪt/	fat cell 脂肪细胞
ana-	up 向上 again 再次	anatomy /ə'nætəmɪ/	cutting up (of the body for study) 解剖
		analysis /ə'næləsɪs/	breaking up (of elements for further understanding) 分析
angi/o	(blood) vessel (血)管	angiitis /ˌəndʒɪ'aɪtɪs/	inflammation of the blood vessel 血管炎，脉管炎
		angioma /ˌændʒɪ'əʊmə/	tumor of the blood vessel 血管瘤
anti-	against 抗	antibiotics /ˌæntɪbaɪ'ɒtɪks/	drug that kills micro-organisms 抗生素
		antidepressant /ˌæntɪdɪ'presənt/	drug that acts against depression 抗抑郁药
bacteri/o	bacterium (pl. bacteria) 细菌	bacteriology /bækˌtɪərɪ'ɒlədʒɪ/	study of bacteria 细菌学
		antibacterial /ˌæntɪbæk 'tɪərɪəl/	acting against bacteria 抗菌的，抗菌药
bi-	two 二，两	bipod /'baɪpɒd/ (*-pod* foot)	two feet 两足，两脚
		bifocal /baɪ'fəʊkəl/	having two foci 双焦点的
-centesis	puncture 穿刺	abdominocentesis /æbˌdɒmɪnəsen'tiːsɪs/	puncture into the abdomen 腹腔穿刺
		arthrocentesis/ɑːˌθrəʊsen'tiːsɪs/ (*arthr/o* joint)	puncture into the joint 关节穿刺
cephal/o	head 头	cephalalgia /ˌsefə'lældʒɪə/	headache 头痛
		cephalic /sɪ'fælɪk/	pertaining to the head 头部的
contra-	opposing 相反 opposite 相对	contraindication /ˌkɒntrəˌɪndɪ'keɪʃən/	medical reasons against certain treatment 禁忌证
		contralateral /ˌkɒntrə'lætərəl/ (*later/o* side)	pertaining to the opposite side 对侧的

Continue

Word Part	Meaning	Example Term	Meaning in English and Chinese
dia-	complete 全 through 贯通	diagnosis /ˌdaɪəg'nəʊsɪs/ (*gn/o* knowledge)	complete knowledge about certain disease 诊断
		diameter /daɪ'æmɪtə/ (*-meter* measure)	measurement of line through the center of a circle 直径
enter/o	small intestine 小肠	enterology /ˌentə'rɒlədʒɪ/	study of small intestine and its diseases 肠病学
		enteritis /ˌentə'raɪtɪs/	inflammation of the small intestine 肠炎
-gram	record 图像 X-ray image 造影片	electrocardiogram /ɪˌlektrəʊ'kɑːdɪəʊgræm/ (*electr/o* electricity)	record of the electric activity of the heart 心电图
		angiogram /'ændʒɪəgram/	X-ray image of the blood vessel 血管造影片
-graph	instrument for recording 记录器，造影仪	chronograph/'krɒnəgrɑːf/ (*chron/o* time)	instrument to record the time 计时器
		electrocardiograph /ɪˌlektrəʊ'kɑːdɪəʊgrɑːf/	instrument to record the electric activity of the heart 心电图机，心电描记器
-graphy	process of recording 描记术，造影术	sonography /sə'nɒgrəfɪ/ (*son/o* sound)	process of recording image by using sound waves 超声描记术
		encephalography /enˌsefə'lɒgrəfɪ/	process of recording the image of the brain 脑造影术
hydr/o	water 水 fluid 液体	dehydration /ˌdiːhaɪ'dreɪʃən/ (*de-* off, separation)	removal of water 脱水
		hydrotherapy /ˌhaɪdrəʊ'θerəpɪ/ (*-therapy* treatment)	treatment using water 水疗
-lysis	breaking down 溶解 separation 分离	hemolysis /hɪ'mɒləsɪs/ (*hem/o* blood)	breaking down of the blood cells 溶血
		electrolysis /ɪˌlek'trɒləsɪs/	separation of chemicals using electricity 电解
neur/o	nerve 神经	neurology /njʊə'rɒlədʒɪ/	study of the nervous system 神经病学
		neuritis /njʊə'raɪtɪs/	inflammation of the nerve 神经炎
-osis	abnormal condition 病态	psychosis /saɪ'kəʊsɪs/ (*psych/o* mind)	abnormal condition of the mind 精神病，精神错乱
		neurosis /njʊə'rəʊsɪs/	abnormal condition of the nerve 神经症
path/o	disease 病	pathology /pə'θɒlədʒɪ/	study of the disease 病理学
		cardiopathy /ˌkɑːdɪ'ɒpəθɪ/	disease of the heart 心脏病
-plasty	surgical repair 外科整形术，成形术	arthroplasty/ˌɑːθrɒ'plæstɪ/	surgical repair of the joint 关节成形术
		angioplasty /'ændʒɪəʊˌplæ stɪ/	surgical repair of the blood vessel 血管成形术
rhin/o, nas/o	nose 鼻	rhinitis /raɪ'naɪtɪs/	inflammation of the nose 鼻炎
		rhinoplasty /'raɪnəʊˌplæ stɪ/	surgical repair of the nose 鼻整形术
		nasal /'neɪzəl/	pertaining to the nose 鼻的
		paranasal /ˌpærə'neɪzəl/ (*para-* near, around)	pertaining to area around the nose 鼻旁的，鼻侧的

Continue

Word Part	Meaning	Example Term	Meaning in English and Chinese
-scope	instrument to view 窥镜	endoscope /'endəskəʊp/	instrument to view the inside of the body 内镜
		microscope /'maɪkrəʊskəʊp/	instrument to view small objects 显微镜
thorac/o	chest 胸部；胸腔	thoracoscope /'θɒrəkəʊskəʊp/	instrument to view the chest 胸腔镜
		thoracic /θɔː'ræsɪk/	pertaining to the chest 胸部的

Exercises

Ⅰ. Decide whether the following statements are true or false. Write T for true and F for false in the blank provided.

__F__ 1. The interpretation of a medical term starts from its prefix.

__T__ 2. If the suffix begins with a vowel, then there is no need for a combining vowel when linking a root with the suffix.

__F__ 3. If the second root begins with a vowel, then a combining vowel is not needed when linking the first root with a second root.

Ⅱ. Use the rule you have learned to build medical terms and explain their meanings. The first one has been provided for you.

1. neur/o + -al = neural, meaning pertaining to nerve
2. rhin/o + -scope = rhinoscope, meaning an instrument to view the nose
3. path/o + -logy = pathology, meaning the study of disease
4. enter/o + -itis = enteritis, meaning inflammation of the small intestine
5. rhin/o + -plasty = rhinoplasty, meaning surgical repair of the nose
6. adip/o + -lysis = adipolysis, meaning breaking down of fat
7. angi/o + -graphy = angiography, meaning process of recording the X-ray image of the blood vessel
8. thorac/o + -centesis = thoracocentesis, meaning puncture into the chest
9. bi- + cephal/o + -ic = bicephalic, meaning pertaining to having two heads
10. electr/o + encephala/o + -gram = electroencephalogram, meaning record of the electric activity of the brain

Ⅲ. Match each word part in Column A with its English meaning in Column B. Write the corresponding letter in the blank provided.

Column A(Word Parts)	Column B(English Terms)
__N__ 1. -plasty	A. small intestine
__E__ 2. -graphy	B. (blood) vessel
__B__ 3. angi/o	C. abnormal condition
__K__ 4. -centesis	D. water, fluid
__A__ 5. enter/o	E. process of recording

Answer	Column A	Column B
O	6. contra-	F. nose
D	7. hydr/o	G. breaking down
C	8. -osis	H. nerve
F	9. rhin/o, nas/o	I. two
M	10. -gram	J. fat
G	11. -lysis	K. puncture
H	12. neur/o	L. head
I	13. bi-	M. record
J	14. adip/o	N. surgical repair
L	15. cephal/o	O. opposing, opposite

Section B Reading Passages

Passage One Human Diseases

Exercises

Ⅰ. Match each term in Column A with its correct description in Column B. Write the corresponding letter in the blank provided.

Answer	Column A	Column B
H	1. abscess	A. a disease transmitted by a specific kind of contact, e.g. cholera
E	2. pathogen	B. a disease that develops and spreads rapidly to many people
J	3. endemic disease	C. carrier
A	4. infectious disease	D. something a patient can detect such as high fever
B	5. epidemic disease	E. any disease-producing agent, like viruses, bacteria and fungi
I	6. chronic disease	F. something a doctor can detect such as high body temperature
C	7. vector	G. inflammation of the lung
D	8. symptom	H. a swelling filled with pus in or on the body
F	9. sign	I. a disease that has a slow onset and runs a long course
G	10. pneumonia	J. a disease that is constantly present in people living in a particular location

Ⅱ. Fill in each blank with one proper word.

A disease is a particular (1) abnormal condition, a disorder of a structure or function that affects part or all of an organism. The causal study of disease is called (2) pathology. Disease is often construed（解释）as a medical condition associated with specific symptoms and (3) signs. It may be caused by factors originally from an (4) external source, such as infectious disease, or it may be caused by internal dysfunctions, such as autoimmune diseases. A (5) pathogen is an infectious agent such as a virus, bacterium, fungus, or parasite that causes disease in its host. Pathogens can rapidly evolve and adapt, and thereby avoid detection by the (6) immune system.

However, multiple defense mechanisms have also evolved to recognize and neutralize（中和）(7) pathogens. Infections with most pathogens do not (8) result in death of the host and the offending organism is ultimately cleared after the symptoms of the diseases have waned. Specific acquired (9) immunity against infectious diseases may be mediated by antibodies and/or T lymphocytes. The immune system response to a microorganism often causes (10) symptoms such as high fever and inflammation, and has the potential to be more devastating than direct damage caused by a microbe.

Ⅲ. Translate the following into English.

1. 功能失调	malfunction	2. 营养不良	malnutrition
3. 致病因子	pathogenic factor	4. 易感人群	vulnerable group
5. 携带者	carrier	6. 病理学	pathology
7. 地方病	endemic disease	8. 病菌	germ
9. 流行病	epidemic disease	10. 感染	infection
11. 吸毒成瘾	drug addiction	12. 吞噬细胞	phagocyte
13. 亚急性疾病	subacute disease	14. 症状	symptom
15. 病原体	pathogen	16. 体征	sign

Ⅳ. Discuss the following topics.

1. What is pathology? What does the modern approach to the study of disorder emphasize?

   Pathology is the science that deals with the structural and functional changes produced by the disease. The modern approach to the study of disorder emphasizes the close relationship of the pathological and physiological aspects and the need to understand the fundamentals of each in treating any body diseases.

2. Describe the classification of diseases.

   Diseases can be classified differently. Epidemic vs. endemic. An epidemic disease is one that strikes many persons in a community. When it strikes the same region year after year, it is an endemic disease. Acute vs. chronic. An acute disease has a quick onset and runs a short course. A chronic disease has a slow onset and runs a sometimes years-long course. Between the acute and chronic, another type is called subacute. Infectious vs. noninfectious. An infectious, or communicable, disease is the one that can be passed between persons such as by means of airborne droplets from a cough or sneeze. Noninfectious diseases are caused by malfunctions of the body.

   Disability and illnesses can also be provoked by psychological and social factors. Furthermore, a thousand or more inheritable birth defects result from alternations in gene patterns.

3. How does the human body fight against diseases?

   The first line of defense is a number of physical barriers, including the skin and mucous membranes, body temperature, wax in the outer ear canals, tears from the eye ducts, and stomach acid. The body's second line of defense is the blood and lymph.

Passage Two Diagnosis and Prognosis

Exercises

Ⅰ. Match each term in Column A with its correct description in Column B. Write the corresponding letter in the blank provided.

Column A	Column B
F 1. chief complaint	A. a graphical record of electric currents associated with muscle contractions
J 2. family history	B. a medical test to determine how quickly glucose is cleared from the blood, and it is usually a test for diabetes
G 3. electrocardiography	C. subsequent examination of a patient for the purpose of monitoring earlier treatment
A 4. electromyogram	D. an estimate about whether a patient will recover from an illness
I 5. spirometer	E. deficiency of healthy red blood cells
H 6. pap smear	F. a patient's statement of what is wrong with him/ her
D 7. prognosis	G. graphical recording of the electric currents associated with contractions of the heart
C 8. follow-up	H. a sample of secretions and superficial cells of the cervix and uterus examined with a microscope to detect abnormal cells
E 9. anemia	I. an instrument for measuring the vital capacity of the lungs
B 10. glucose-tolerance test	J. part of a medical history in which questions are asked to find out whether the patient has hereditary tendencies toward particular diseases

Ⅱ. Fill in each blank with a correct term in the box. Change the form of the words if necessary.

sequela	immunization	allergy	biopsy
hospitalization	symptom	microorganism	degenerative
mammography	anemia	pulmonary	

1. Cases of major burns require medical treatment and hospitalization.
2. Immunization is the process by which an individual's immune system becomes strengthened against an agent.
3. Food allergies can result in an enormous variety of symptoms, for example, nausea, vomiting, abdominal pain and itching skin.

4. I like cats but unfortunately, I'm allergic to animal hair.
5. Anemia is usually defined as a decrease in the amount of red blood cells or hemoglobin in the blood.
6. A microorganism is a very small living thing which you can only see if you use a microscope.
7. A biopsy is the medical removal of tissue from a living subject to determine the presence or extent of a disease.
8. The woman was taking an X-ray examination of her breast for tumor, a procedure called mammography.
9. Chronic kidney disease is sometimes a sequela of diabetes.
10. The primary purpose of pulmonary function testing is to identify the severity of lung impairment.

Ⅲ. Translate the following sentences into Chinese.

1. Since body fluids often reveal important information about the nature of the disorder, laboratory testing plays an important role in determining the patient's disease.
   由于体液常常揭示了关于疾病性质的重要信息，所以实验室检查对于确诊疾病起着重要的作用。
2. Mucus from the nose and throat can be tested to identify the organisms responsible for respiratory infections.
   鼻腔和喉部的黏液检查常常可用于确定引起呼吸道感染的微生物。
3. Nuclear magnetic resonance, or magnetic resonance imaging, is a hazard-free, non-invasive method that uses radio waves in the presence of a strong magnetic field to probe a patient and generate visual images of thin slices of the brain, heart, liver, and other organs.
   核磁共振（即磁共振成像）是一种无副作用、无创的检查方法，运用强磁场下的无线电波来对患者进行检查，并生成脑、心脏、肝脏及其他器官的薄层可视图像。
4. Mammography, a procedure that involves using special X-rays to produce an image of the soft tissues of the breast, is a much more reliable way to detect tumors.
   乳腺 X 线照相术使用特殊的 X 射线产生乳房的软组织图像，是一种更可靠的检测肿瘤的方法。
5. The best physicians blend honest fact and hope together, helping the patient through the complicated steps of shock, denial, depression, and acceptance of fatal illness.
   最高明的医生在告知病人事实时也会给予希望，帮助病人走出震惊、否定、抑郁的复杂情绪，并最终接受绝症这一事实。

Ⅳ. Discuss the following topics.

1. Suppose you are facing a group of physicians who come from a rural area in China for in-service training. Tell them what should be included as the major content in a medical history.
   A medical history mainly includes the following contents: description of the patient, chief complaints, other physicians involved in the patient's care, history of the present illness, past medical history, social and occupational history, family history, and review of systems.

2. Give a brief account of three laboratory tests mentioned in the passage.
   The answer is open.
3. Why is the handling of prognosis important both for doctors and patients?
   The answer is open.

Passage Three Approach to the Patient

Exercises

I. Choose the best answer to each of the following questions.

1. What is the correct attitude a doctor should assume in coping with the "Five D's" of a patient? __B__
   A. Trying his best first and then giving up if there is no hope.
   B. Keeping on trying though he might fail.
   C. Continuing to try till meeting his failure.
   D. Keeping on trying and never admitting failure.
2. Which one is a right principle of treatment? __C__
   A. The top task of the physician is to treat the disease.
   B. Relieving symptoms is less important than tackling infection.
   C. The patient's participation can influence the success of a treatment.
   D. Only treatment can improve the health of a patient.
3. The major purpose of signing consent before a therapeutic procedure is to __D__.
   A. prevent legal dispute between the patient and the doctor
   B. protect the doctor's rights in case of a medical accident
   C. give professional advice to the patient and make the final decision for them
   D. ensure that the patient has a thorough understanding about the procedure before making the final decision
4. The sentence "the physician should act as the patient's advocate" means __B__.
   A. the physician should support the patient's idea of seeking medical treatment
   B. the physician should speak on behalf of the patient's interest
   C. the physician should advocate the idea he thinks the patient should follow
   D. the physician should purposely speak the opposite of what a patient might say
5. When giving medications to the patient, it is important that __A__.
   A. the doctor should explain the purpose, the dosage and the course of the medication
   B. the doctor should conceal the side effects of the medication so that the patient will be more willing to cooperate
   C. the patient should remember the names of the medications
   D. the patient should not take the medications prescribed by more than one doctor at the same time
6. Which one is a correct rule for helping patients take prescribed medication? __D__
   A. Prescribing no more than two kinds of medications each time.

B. Prescribing the least expensive medication with the simplest dosage schedule.

C. Never changing the medication at the follow-up visits.

D. Writing down instructions to help those who have trouble remembering to take medicines.

7. According to the passage, prevention and health maintenance involve __B__.

A. regular exercises, balanced diet, and sound sleep

B. screening examinations, immunizations and lifestyle counseling

C. not taking medicine when having mild ailments

D. going to hospital regularly for checking-up

8. If the patient fails to make a lifestyle change, the doctor should __C__.

A. concentrate on the actual steps the patient should take

B. advise the patient to do screening tests

C. encourage the patient to keep trying

D. criticize the patient and change the plan

9. A physician has to do a great deal of synthesis and judgment because he/she must __A__.

A. be considering many different elements at once

B. think of the diagnostic possibilities and the prognostic implications

C. consider what he/she should say to the patient and how to say it

D. think of which laboratory tests and therapy to choose and how to explain them to the patient

Ⅱ. Here is a list of terms from the text. Analyze their meanings using the word building knowledge you have learned. Leave the space empty if the word part does not apply.

Term	Prefix	Combining Form/Root	Suffix	Chinese Translation
1. premature	pre-	mature		过早的
2. angioplasty		angi/o	-plasty	血管成形术
3. mammogram		mamm/o	-gram	乳腺X线照片
4. asymptomatic	a-	symptom	-tic	无症状的
5. immunization		immun/o	-ize -ation	预防接种
6. discomfort	dis-	comfort		不适
7. chemotherapy	chemo-	therapy		化疗

Chapter Three Muscular System

 Section A Medical Terminology

Learn the following combining forms, prefixes and suffixes for the muscular system and write the meanings of the medical terms in the space provided.

Word Part	Meaning	Example Term	Meaning in English and Chinese
ab-	away from 脱离；离开	abductor /æb'dʌktə/	a muscle that draws a body part away from the median line 外展肌
		aboral /æ'bɔːrəl/	away from or opposite the mouth 离口的；对口的
ad-	toward 朝着；向	adrenal /æd'riːnəl/ (*ren/o* kidney)	on or near the kidneys 肾上的；肾旁的
		adductor /ə'dʌktə/	a muscle that draws a body part toward the median line 内收肌
ante-	forward, front 前；前面	anteflexion /ˌæntə'flekʃən/ (*flex/o* bending)	bending forward 前屈
		anterior /æn'tɪərɪə/	toward the front 前部的
brachi/o	arm 手臂	brachiocephalic /ˌbrækɪəʊsə'fælɪk/	pertaining to the arm and head 头臂的
		brachialgia /ˌbrækɪ'ældʒɪə/	pain of the arm 臂痛
-ceps	points of muscle attachment 肌头	biceps /'baɪseps/	a two-headed muscle 二头肌
		triceps /'traɪseps/	a three-headed muscle 三头肌
-desis	binding 固定术	myodesis /maɪ'əʊdiːsɪs/	binding of the muscle 肌肉固定术
		arthrodesis /ˌɑːθrəʊ'diːsɪs/	binding of the joint 关节固定术
-dynia	pain 疼痛	neurodynia /ˌnjʊərə'dɪnɪə/	pain of the nerve 神经痛
		arthrodynia /'ɑːθrəˌdɪnɪə/	pain of the joint 关节疼痛
fibr/o	fiber 纤维	fibrosis /faɪ'brəʊsɪs/	abnormal growth of the fiber tissue 纤维化
		fibrocyte /'faɪbrəʊsaɪt/	fiber cell 纤维细胞
-kinesis	movement 运动	akinesis /'eɪkɪˌniːsɪs/	loss of movement 运动失能
		dyskinesis /ˌdɪskɪ'niːsɪs/	having difficulty in movement 运动障碍
morph/o	shape 形状；形态	polymorphic /ˌpɒlɪ'mɔːfɪk/ (*poly-* many)	having many shapes 多形态的，不定形的
		morphology /mɔː'fɒlədʒɪ/	study of the shape (of cells) 形态学

Continue

Word Part	Meaning	Example Term	Meaning in English and Chinese
my/o musculo/o	muscle 肌肉	myotomy /maɪ'ɒtəmɪ/	incision into the muscle 肌切开术
		myolysis /maɪ'ɒlɪsɪs/	breaking down of the muscle 肌肉溶解
		muscular /'mʌskjuːlə/	pertaining to the muscle 肌的
		intramuscular /ˌɪntrə'mʌskjuːlə/ (*intra-* within)	within the muscle 肌内的
-oma	tumor（肿）瘤 mass 肿块	myoma /maɪ'əʊmə/	tumor of the muscle 肌瘤
		neuroma /njʊə'rəʊmə/	tumor of the nerve 神经瘤
-pathy	disease 病	myopathy /maɪ'ɒpəθɪ/	disease of the muscle 肌病
		cardiopathy /ˌkaːdɪ'ɒpəθɪ/	disease of the heart 心脏病
-rrhaphy	surgical suture 缝合术	myorrhaphy /maɪ'ɒrəfɪ/	surgical suture of the muscle 肌缝合术
		herniorrhaphy /ˌhɜːnɪ'ɔːrəfɪ/ (*herni/o* hernia)	surgical suture of the hernia 疝缝合术
-rrhexia, -rrhexis	rupture 破裂	hepatorrhexia /ˌhepətəʊ'reksɪə/	rupture of the liver 肝脏破裂
		myorrhexis /ˌmaɪəʊ'reksɪs/	rupture of the muscle 肌断裂
sarc/o	flesh 肉	sarcoma /saː'kəʊmə/	fleshy tumor 肉瘤
		sarcolysis /saː'kɒlɪsɪs/	breaking down of the flesh 肌肉分解，软组织分解
-spasm	involuntary contraction 痉挛	enterospasm /'entərəˌspæzəm/	involuntary contraction of the small intestine 肠痉挛
		myospasm/'maɪɒˌspæzəm/	involuntary contraction of the muscle 肌肉痉挛
ten/o, tendin/o	tendon 肌腱	tenoplasty /ˌtenə'plæstɪ/	surgical repair of the tendon 腱成形术
		tenalgia /te'nældʒɪə/	pain of the tendon 腱痛
		tendinorrhaphy /ˌtendɪ'nɒrəfɪ/	surgical suture of the tendon 腱缝合术
		tendinitis /ˌtendɪ'naɪtɪs/	inflammation of the tendon 肌腱炎
ton/o	tension 张力 pressure 压力	dystonia /dɪs'təʊnɪə/	abnormal tension（肌）张力失常
		atonia /ə'təʊnɪə/	lack of tension 张力缺乏
troph/o	nourishment 营养	atrophy /'ætrəfɪ/	decrease of cells in size due to lack of nourishment 萎缩
		hypertrophy/'haɪpɜːˌtrəʊfɪ/	increase of cells in size due to excessive nourishment 肥大

Exercises

Ⅰ. Fill in the following blanks with the terms in the box.

tenorrhexia	trophopathy
biceps	dystonia
intramuscular	dyskinesis
amorphous	tenoplasty

1. Something that is amorphous has no clear shape or structure.
2. A patient suffers from dyskinesis has difficulty in carrying out movement.
3. An athlete tore his tendon during a football match, a medical condition known as tenorrhexia, and was sent to a hospital for an emergency surgery to repair the ruptured tendon. The surgery is also called tenoplasty.
4. A(n) intramuscular injection is a shot of medicine injected into the muscle for absorption.
5. Both overweight and underweight are disorders related to nutrition. The medical term for the disease related to abnormality of nutrition is trophopathy.
6. Brain infection can lead to dystonia, abnormal tension of the muscle, in which patients have difficulty controlling their postures and voluntary movement.
7. The large muscles at the front of the upper part of your arms have two points of attachment; hence, they are called biceps.

Ⅱ. Write a word for each of the following definitions.

1. tumor of the muscle — myoma
2. involuntary contraction of the muscle — myospasm
3. abnormal nourishment of the muscle — myodystrophy
4. slow (*brady-*) movement — bradykinesis
5. front of the arm, forearm — antebrachium
6. surgical suture of the tendon — tendinorrhaphy
7. a muscle cell — myocyte
8. excessive (*hyper-*) tension — hypertonia
9. disease of the tendon — tendinopathy
10. a four (*quadr/i*) headed muscle — quadriceps

Ⅲ. Match each word part in Column A with its English term in Column B. Write the corresponding letter in the blank provided.

	Column A	Column B
H	1. fibr/o	A. binding
J	2. -kinesis	B. flesh
A	3. -desis	C. nourishment
G	4. -spasm	D. muscle
B	5. sarc/o	E. forward
D	6. muscul/o	F. tendon
C	7. troph/o	G. involuntary contraction
E	8. ante-	H. fiber
I	9. brachi/o	I. arm
F	10. ten/o, tendin/o	J. movement

Section B Reading Passages

Passage One Muscles

Exercises

Ⅰ. Match each term in Column A with its correct description in Column B. Write the corresponding letter in the blank provided.

Column A	Column B
D 1. skeletal muscle	A. decrease in size of an organ caused by disease or disuse
A 2. atrophy	B. specialized bit of heart tissue that controls the heartbeat
E 3. tendon	C. of or involving the arteries
F 4. willpower	D. muscle that is connected at either or both ends to a bone and so moves parts of the skeleton
J 5. hypertrophy	E. a cord or band of inelastic tissue connecting a muscle with its bony attachment
I 6. contraction	F. the trait of resolutely controlling your own behavior
B 7. sinoatrial node	G. skeletal muscle whose contraction extends or stretches a body part
C 8. arterial	H. painful and involuntary muscular contraction
G 9. extensor	I. shortening or tensing of a part or organ (especially of a muscle or muscle fiber)
H 10. cramp	J. abnormal enlargement of a body part or organ

Ⅱ. Fill in each blank with one proper word.

Muscle tissue is a (1) soft tissue, and is one of the four fundamental types of tissue present in animals. The three types of muscle tissue are cardiac, (2) smooth, and skeletal. (3) Cardiac muscle cells are located in the walls of the heart, appear striated, and are under (4) involuntary control. (5) Smooth muscle fibers are located in walls of hollow visceral organs, except the heart, appear spindle-shaped, and are also under involuntary control. Smooth muscle is responsible for the (6) contractility of hollow organs, such as blood vessels, the gastrointestinal tract, the bladder, or the uterus. Skeletal muscle fibers are present in muscles which are attached to the (7) skeleton. They are (8) striated in appearance and are under voluntary control. They are usually connected to the skeletal system by bundles of collagen fibers which are more commonly known as (9) tendons. The point at which the muscle attaches to the bone is called the (10) origin of the muscle.

Ⅲ. Translate the following into English.

1. 肌纤维 muscle fiber
2. 随意肌 voluntary muscle
3. 消化道 alimentary canal
4. 肌腹 muscle belly
5. 横纹肌 striated muscle
6. 肌肉肥大 muscle hypertrophy

7. 肌肉收缩	muscle contraction	8. 肌肉附着点	attachment of the muscle
9. 肌肉放松	muscle relaxation	10. 肌腱	tendon
11. 止端	insertion	12. 起端	origin
13. 伸肌	extensor	14. 屈肌	flexor
15. 横切面	transverse section	16. 纤维结缔组织	fibrous connective tissue

Ⅳ. Discuss the following topics.

1. What is the difference between voluntary and involuntary muscles?
   Voluntary muscles are under the control of our willpower while involuntary muscles are not controlled by our willpower.
2. What is the difference between striated and nonstriated muscles?
   When viewed under a microscope, striated muscles have cross striations of the muscle fibers whereas there is no striation presented in nonstriated muscles.
3. Give a brief account of the functions of skeletal, smooth and cardiac muscles, respectively.
   Skeletal muscles help hold the bones of the skeleton together and give the body shape; they also make the body move. Smooth muscles often make the walls of blood vessels and the alimentary canal; they are usually found as a sheath of muscle fibers surrounding a tube-like structure. Coordinated contractions of cardiac muscle cells in the heart propel blood out of the atria and ventricles to the blood vessels of the circulatory systems.

Passage Two Common Muscle Disorders and Diseases

Exercises

Ⅰ. Match each term in Column A with its correct description in Column B. Write the corresponding letter in the blank provided.

	Column A	Column B
D	1. myositis	A. an expected time to live as calculated on the basis of statistical probabilities
H	2. toxin	B. the bony arch formed by the collarbones and shoulder blades in humans
G	3. atrophy	C. any visible abnormal structural change in a bodily part
F	4. dystrophy	D. inflammation of muscle tissue
J	5. myasthenia gravis	E. origination and development of a disease
I	6. paralysis	F. any degenerative disorder resulting from inadequate or faulty nutrition
B	7. shoulder girdle	G. decrease in size of an organ caused by disease or disuse
E	8. pathogenesis	H. a poisonous substance
A	9. life expectancy	I. loss of the ability to move a body part
C	10. lesion	J. chronic progressive disease characterized by chronic fatigue and muscular weakness

Ⅱ. Fill in each blank with a correct term in the box. Change the form of the words if necessary.

muscle fatigue	neuromuscular	myositis	contraction
muscular dystrophy	musculoskeletal	limb-girdle muscular dystrophy	
muscle soreness	atrophy	Duchenne muscular dystrophy	

1. Muscle soreness is the pain and stiffness felt in muscles several hours to days after unaccustomed or strenuous exercise.
2. Skeletal muscle cramps may be caused by any combination of muscle fatigue and a lack of electrolytes (e.g., low sodium, low potassium, or low magnesium).
3. Myasthenia gravis is a neuromuscular disease that leads to muscle weakness and fatigue.
4. Myositis is a general term for inflammation of the muscles.
5. Duchenne muscular dystrophy is a recessive X-linked form of muscular dystrophy, affecting around 1 in 3,600 boys, which results in muscle degeneration and premature death.
6. A cramp is a sudden and involuntary muscle contraction.
7. Muscular dystrophies are characterized by progressive skeletal muscle weakness, defects in muscle proteins, and the death of muscle cells and tissue.
8. A muscle becomes atrophied when its fibers get smaller and its total size decreases.
9. Muscular dystrophy is a group of muscle diseases that weaken the musculoskeletal system and hamper locomotion.
10. Limb-girdle muscular dystrophy is characterized by progressive muscle wasting which affects predominantly hip and shoulder muscles.

Ⅲ. Translate the following sentences into Chinese.

1. Muscle atrophy is an acquired lesion secondary to some well-defined predisposing cause; muscular dystrophy refers to a variety of genetically determined primary disorders of muscles.
肌萎缩是继发于某些明确素因性原因的获得性病变，而肌营养不良则指多种原发的遗传性肌肉病变。
2. Muscular dystrophies must be distinguished from congenital myopathies, which are characterized by fairly specific distinctive morphologic changes.
必须将肌营养不良与先天性肌病相区别，后者呈鲜明的形态学改变。
3. Myasthenia gravis is a relapsing, remitting neuromuscular disorder characterized by weakness and pronounced fatigability of the skeletal muscles.
重症肌无力是一种反复发作的神经肌肉疾病，其特征是骨骼肌无力及明显的易疲倦。
4. The muscular dystrophies are traditionally subdivided according to the patterns of initial muscle involvement, which in turn correlated fairly well with the type of genetic transmission.
肌营养不良传统上依据其初始受累的肌肉情况再分为几个亚型，这与基因传递的类型相当吻合。
5. Inflammatory myositis may also be encountered in many of the so-called connective tissue diseases, most of which are believed to be immunologic in origin.
某些结缔组织病也可能出现感染性肌炎，这些疾病大多被认为源于免疫系统。

Ⅳ. Discuss the following topics.

1. List three of the common muscle disorders and diseases.
   Three common muscle disorders are muscle soreness, cramp and muscle fatigue. Three common muscle diseases are muscle atrophy, muscular dystrophy and myasthenia gravis.
2. As a linguist, how would you explain the difference between muscle atrophy and dystrophy? As a physician, how would you explain the difference between muscle atrophy and dystrophy?
   The answer is open.
3. What are the three major patterns of muscular dystrophies?
   The three major patterns are Duchenne (pseudohypertrophic) muscular dystrophy, limb girdle muscular dystrophy and facioscapulohumeral muscular dystrophy.

Passage Three Muscular Dystrophy

Exercises

Ⅰ. Read the following statements and decide whether they are true or false. Then write T for true and F for false in the brackets.

1. [F] Neurologist Guillaume Duchenne was the first to report on muscular dystrophy.
2. [T] Muscular dystrophy can affect both boys and girls.
3. [F] Certain forms of muscular dystrophies are caused by muscle injury.
4. [F] Boys are at a greater risk of inheriting the defective gene from their parents.
5. [T] For a girl, the faulty X chromosome received from her mother can be offset by the healthy one she receives from her father.
6. [F] Duchenne muscular dystrophy cases always have prior family history.
7. [F] Approximately 1 in every 3,500 to 6,000 children is affected by Duchenne muscular dystrophy in the United States.
8. [F] Autosomal recessive inheritance means a child receives a normal gene from one parent and a defective gene from the other parent.
9. [F] Muscular dystrophy can be prevented and reversed with proper treatment.
10. [T] The goal of available treatments is to help MD patients live a longer and better life.

Ⅱ. Here is a list of terms from the text. Analyze their meanings using the word building knowledge you have learned. Leave the space empty if the word part does not apply.

Term	Prefix	Combining Form/Root	Suffix	Chinese Translation
1. tuberculosis		tubercul/o	-sis	肺结核
2. neurologist		neur/o	-logist	神经病学家
3. phagocytosis		phag/o cyt/o	-sis	噬菌作用
4. gastrointestinal		gastr/o interstin/o	-al	胃肠的
5. glycoprotein		glyc/o protein		糖蛋白
6. prenatal	pre-	nat/o	-al	产前的
7. dystrophy	dys-	troph/o	-y	营养不良

Chapter Four Skeletal System

Section A Medical Terminology

Learn the following combining forms, prefixes and suffixes for the skeletal system and write the meanings of the medical terms in the space provided.

Word Part	Meaning	Example Term	Meaning in English and Chinese
arthr/o, articul/o	joint 关节	arthrodesis /ˌɑːθrəʊ'diːsɪs/	binding of the joint 关节固定术
		arthrotomy /ɑː'θrəʊtəmɪ/	incision into the joint 关节切开术
		biarticular /baɪə'tɪkjʊlə/	pertaining to two joints 双关节的
		circumarticular /ˌsɜːkəmɑː'tɪkjʊlə/ (*circum*-surrounding)	surrounding the joint 关节周的
-blast	embryonic cell 胚细胞 immature cell 成……细胞	neuroblast /'njʊərəblæst/	immature nerve cell 成神经细胞
		osteoblast /'ɒstɪəblæst/ (*oste/o* bone)	immature bone cell 成骨细胞
calc/i	calcium 钙	calcipenia /ˌkælsɪ'piːnɪə/ (*-penia* deficiency)	calcium deficiency 钙缺乏
		calcify /'kælsɪfaɪ/	to become calcium 钙化
cervic/o	neck 颈	cervicodorsal /ˌsɜːvɪkəʊ'dɔːsəl/ (*dors/o* back)	pertaining to the neck and back 颈背的
		cervicodynia /ˌsɜːvɪkəʊ'dɪnɪə/	pain of the neck 颈痛
chondr/o	cartilage 软骨	chondroblastoma /ˌkɒndrɒblɑː'stəʊmə/	tumor of the immature cartilage 成软骨细胞瘤
		chondrocyte /'kʌdrɒsaɪt/	cartilage cell 软骨细胞
-clast	breaking cell 破……细胞	osteoclast /'ɒstɪəʊklæst/	bone-breaking cell 破骨细胞
		chondroclast /ˌkɒndrəʊ'klæst/	cartilage-breaking cell 破软骨细胞
cost/o	rib 肋	costectomy /kɒ'stektəmɪ/	excision of the rib 肋骨切除术
		costalgia /kɒ'stældʒɪə/	pain of the rib 肋痛
crani/o	skull 颅骨	cranioplasty /ˌkreɪnɪəʊ'plæstɪ/	surgical repair of the skull 颅成形术
		craniocervical /ˌkreɪnɪəʊ'sɜːveɪkəl/	pertaining to the skull and neck 颅颈的

Continue

Word Part	Meaning	Example Term	Meaning in English and Chinese
dent/o, odont/o	tooth 牙齿	dentist /ˈdentɪst/	a specialist in treating teeth 牙科医生
		dental /ˈdentəl/	pertaining to teeth 牙(科)的
		odontoneuralgia /ˌɒdɒntəʊnjʊəˈræl dʒɪə/	pain of the nerve in the tooth 牙神经痛
		periodontitis /ˌperɪɒdɒnˈtaɪtɪs/ (*peri-* around)	inflammation around the tooth 牙周炎
femor/o	femur 股骨	femoro-articular /ˌfemərəʊɑːˈtɪkjʊlə/	pertaining to the femur and joint 股骨关节的
		femoral /ˈfemərəl/	pertaining to the femur 股骨的
gnath/o	jaw 颌骨	dysgnathia /dɪsgˈnæθɪə/	abnormal jaw development 颌发育不良
		gnathoplasty /ˈnæθəʊˌplæstɪ/	surgical repair of the jaw 颌成形术
ili/o	ilium 髂骨	iliocostal /ˌɪlɪəˈkɒstəl/	pertaining to the ilium and rib 髂肋的
		iliofemoral /ˌɪlɪəˈfemərəl/	pertaining to the ilium and femur 髂股的
inter-	between 之间	inter-articular /ˌɪntəɑːˈtɪkjʊlə/	between the joints 关节间的
		intercostal /ˌɪntəˈkɒstəl/	between the ribs 肋间的
intra-	inner, inside 内	intrachondrial /ˌɪntrəˈkɒndrɪəl/	inside the cartilage 软骨内的
		intracranial /ˌɪntrəˈkreɪnɪəl/	inside the skull 颅内的
-malacia	softening 软化	craniomalacia /ˌkreɪnɪɒməˈleɪʃɪə/	softening of the cranium 颅骨软化
		chondromalacia /ˌkɒndrəʊməˈleɪʃɪə/	softening of the cartilage 软骨软化
orth/o	straight 正；直	orthognathia /ˌɔːθɒgˈneɪθɪə/	straightening of the jaw 正颌
		orthodontics /ˌɔːθəˈdɒntɪks/	straightening of the tooth 正齿
oste/o	bone 骨	osteopathy /ˌɒstɪˈɒpəθɪ/	disease of the bone 骨病
		osteomalacia /ˌɒstɪəʊməˈleɪʃɪə/	softening of the bone 骨软化
pelv/i	pelvis 骨盆	pelvimetry /pelˈvɪmɪtrɪ/ (*-metry* measuring)	measuring of the pelvis 骨盆测量
		intrapelvic /ˌɪntrəˈpelvɪk/	inside the pelvis 骨盆内的
-um	structure 结构 substance 物质	cranium /ˈkreɪnɪəm/	skull 颅骨
		calcium /ˈkælsɪəm/	lime 钙；石灰
vertebr/o	spine, vertebra 脊椎	intervertebral /ˌɪntəˈvɜːtɪbrəl/	between the spines 椎间的
		intravertebral /ˌɪntrəˈvɜːtɪbrəl/	inside the spine 椎管内的

Exercises

Ⅰ. Fill in the following blanks with the terms in the box.

periodontitis	osteoclast
intercostal	calcium
intracranial	osteoblast
orthodontist	arthropathy

1. Nowadays, the artificial joint replacement surgery has become the standard procedure in treating severe arthropathy.
2. Periodontitis is an advanced form of gum disease resulting in inflammation of the supporting tissues of the teeth.
3. Vitamin D helps the body absorb calcium and stimulates bone formation.
4. During exhalation, your diaphragm and the muscles between your ribs, also known as intercostal muscles, relax, making the chest cavity smaller. The pressure goes up and air rushes out.
5. The cells that synthesize bones are called osteoblasts, while cells that break down bones are known as osteoclasts.
6. In traumatic brain injury, it is very important to monitor the intracranial pressure of the patient. Any elevation of the pressure might lead to secondary brain damage.
7. Today it is relatively rare for someone to have perfectly straight teeth without having been to an orthodontist.

Ⅱ. Write the English and Chinese meanings of the following terms.

1. chondroma tumor of the cartilage 软骨瘤
2. abdominopelvic pertaining to the abdomen and pelvis 腹盆腔的
3. vertebrocostal pertaining to the spine and rib 脊椎肋骨的
4. osteoarthritis inflammation of the bone and joint 骨关节炎
5. craniomalacia softening of the cranium 颅骨软化
6. micrognathia small jaw 小颌(畸形)
7. odontoblast immature tooth cell 成牙质细胞
8. intra-articular inside the joint 关节内的
9. chondrocyte cartilage cell 软骨细胞
10. interdental between the teeth 齿间的

Ⅲ. Match each word part in Column A with its English term in Column B. Write the corresponding letter in the blank provided.

Column A	Column B
C 1. inter-	A. tooth
H 2. -um	B. jaw
D 3. orth/o	C. between

G	4. vertebr/o	D. straight
F	5. oste/o	E. cartilage
J	6. -malacia	F. bone
E	7. chondr/o	G. spine
I	8. cost/o	H. structure, substance
A	9. odont/o	I. rib
B	10. gnath/o	J. softening

Section B Reading Passages

Passage One The Skeletal System

Exercises

Ⅰ. Match each term in Column A with its correct description in Column B. Write the corresponding letter in the blank provided.

	Column A	Column B
B	1. vertebra	A. the fatty network of connective tissue that fills the cavities of bones
H	2. parathormone	B. one of the bony segments of the spinal column
G	3. kneecap	C. the part of the skull that encloses the brain
E	4. homatopoiesis	D. abnormal loss of bony tissue resulting in fragile porous bones attributable to a lack of calcium
J	5. phalanx	E. production and development of blood cells, normally in the bone marrow
I	6. ossification	F. process in which organic tissue becomes hardened by the deposition of lime salts in the tissues
A	7. marrow	G. a small flat triangular bone in front of the knee that protects the knee joint
F	8. calcification	H. hormone secreted by the parathyroid glands
D	9. osteoporosis	I. the developmental process of bone formation
C	10. cranium	J. the bones of the fingers

Ⅱ. Fill in each blank with one proper word or phrase.

The skeleton system serves several basic functions: (1) support, movement, protection, production of (2) blood cells, and storage of minerals. The (3) long bones are those that are longer than they are wide. They are one of four types of bones: long, (4) short, flat, and irregular. The long bones of the human (5) leg comprise nearly half of adult height. Short bones are designated as those bones that are as (6) wide as they are long. Flat bones are bones whose principal function is either extensive (7) protection or the provision of broad surfaces for muscular (8) attachment.

The (9) irregular bones are ones which, from their peculiar form, cannot be grouped as long bone, short bone or flat bone. Bone growth in length is stimulated by the production of (10) growth hormone, a secretion of the anterior lobe of the pituitary gland.

Ⅲ. Translate the following into English.

1. 矿物质吸收	mineral absorption	2. 骨化	ossification
3. 机械应力	mechanical stress	4. 骨钙丧失	loss of calcium from bones
5. 骨基质	bone matrix	6. 生长激素	growth hormone
7. 骨骼系统	skeletal system	8. 骺软骨	epiphyseal cartilage
9. 软骨内骨化	endochondral ossification	10. 降钙素	calcitonin
11. 肋骨架	rib cage	12. 髌骨	patella
13. 松质骨	spongy bone	14. 密质骨	compact bone
15. 骨折	fracture	16. 骨髓腔	marrow cavity
17. 不规则骨	irregular bone	18. 红骨髓	red marrow

Ⅳ. Discuss the following topics.

1. Suppose you were a lecturer of anatomy, please illustrate the functions of the skeletal system.
   One of the main functions of the skeletal system involves providing support for the body and protection for its internal organs. Joints and muscles are connected to bones, making them essential for movement. Minerals are stored here and then distributed to other parts of the body on demand. Blood cells are produced in the skeletal system.
2. Give a brief account of each type of the bones.
   Long bones have greater length than width and consist of a diaphysis and a variable number of epiphyses; they are slightly curved for strength. Short bones are somewhat cube-shaped and nearly equal in length and width. Flat bones are generally thin and composed of two more or less parallel plates of compact bone enclosing a layer of spongy bone. Irregular bones have complex shapes and cannot be grouped into any of the three categories just described.
3. Why are vitamins and minerals important in bone replacement?
   Because calcium and phosphorus are the components of the primary salt that makes bone hard. Manganese is also important in bone growth. It has been shown that manganese deficiency significantly inhibits laying down new bone tissue. Vitamins, particularly vitamin D, participate in the absorption of calcium from the gastrointestinal tract into the blood, calcium removal from bone, and the kidney's reabsorption of calcium that might otherwise be lost in urine.

Passage Two　Disorders of Bones and Joints

Exercises

Ⅰ. Define the types of fractures in the space given below.

1. closed fracture　A simple fracture with no open wound.
2. open fracture　A fracture which is associated with an open wound, or a broken bone protruding through the skin.

3. transverse fracture A break at right angles to the long axis of a bone.
4. spiral fracture A fracture which is in a spiral or S shape, usually caused by twisting injuries.
5. comminuted fracture A fracture in which the bone is splintered or crushed.
6. impacted fracture One fragment is driven into the other.
7. greenstick fracture One side of the bone is broken and the other side is bent.
8. oblique frature A break occurs at an angle across the bone.

Ⅱ. Fill in each blank with a correct term in the box. Change the form of the words if necessary.

transverse	tumor	uric acid	comminuted	fracture
inflammation	rheumatoid	pain	osteomyelitis	cartilage

1. A bone fracture is a medical condition in which there is a damage in the continuity of the bone.
2. Chondrosarcoma is a cancer composed of cells derived from transformed cells that produce cartilage.
3. A transverse fracture is a specific type of broken bone where the break is at a right angle to the long plane of the bone.
4. An osteosarcoma is a cancerous tumor in a bone.
5. Gout is caused by elevated levels of uric acid in the blood.
6. Comminuted fracture is very unstable. The bone shatters into three or more pieces.
7. Arthritis is a form of joint disorder that involves inflammation of one or more joints.
8. The most common symptom of bone tumors is pain, which will gradually increase over time. Additional symptoms may include fatigue, fever, weight loss, anemia（贫血）, and unexplained bone fractures.
9. Osteomyelitis is infection and inflammation of the bone or bone marrow.
10. Rheumatoid arthritis is a disorder in which the body's own immune system starts to attack body tissues. The attack is not only directed at the joint but to many other parts of the body.

Ⅲ. Translate the following sentences into Chinese.

1. Osteomyelitis is an inflammation of bone caused by pus-forming bacteria that enter through a wound or are carried by the blood.
骨髓炎是由进入伤口或血液的化脓性细菌引起的骨骼感染。
2. The effects of a fracture depend on the location and severity of the break, the amount of associated injury, possible complications, such as infections, and success of healing, which may take months.
骨折的预后与断裂部位、严重程度、周围组织损伤程度、可能的并发症(如感染)以及愈合成功与否有关。
3. Osteoarthritis usually appears at midlife and beyond and involves the weight-bearing joints

and joints of the fingers.

骨关节炎通常发生于中老年人，常累及负重关节及手指关节。

4. Osteoporosis may also be caused by nutritional deficiencies, disuse, as in paralysis or immobilization in a cast, and excess steroids from the adrenal cortex.

   骨质疏松症同样可由营养缺乏、因瘫痪或石膏制动而致的废用以及肾上腺皮质分泌类固醇过量等引起。

5. Signs of bone tumors are pain, easy fracture, and increases in serum calcium and alkaline phosphatase.

   骨肿瘤的表现为疼痛、易骨折、血清中钙和碱性磷酸酶含量增高。

Ⅳ. Discuss the following topics.

1. What parts of the bone are commonly affected by an infection?

   The blood-rich ends of the long bones are often invaded by pus-forming bacteria, and the infection then spreads to other regions, such as the bone marrow and even the joints.

2. Give a brief account of metabolic bone diseases.

   Osteoporosis is a loss of bone mass that results in weakening of the bones. A decline in estrogen after menopause makes women over 50 most susceptible to this disorder. In osteomalacia there is a softening of bone tissue due to lack of formation of a calcium salts. Paget disease (osteitis deformans) is a disorder of aging in which bones become larger but weaker. It usually involves the bones of the axial skeleton, causing pain, fractures and hearing loss.

3. What is the difference between osteogenic sarcoma and chondrosarcoma?

   Osteogenic sarcoma most commonly occurs in the growing region of a bone, especially around the knee. Chondrosarcoma usually appears in midlife; as the name implies, this tumor arises in cartilage.

Passage Three　Osteoarthritis

Exercises

Ⅰ. Read the following statements and decide whether they are true or false. Then write T for true and F for false in the brackets.

1. [F] Cartilage is the soft and slippery tissue that protects our joints.
2. [T] Osteoarthritis affects only our joints.
3. [F] Osteoarthritis affects our joints symmetrically.
4. [F] Osteoarthritis does not affect younger people.
5. [F] Osteoarthritis is more common in women than in men.
6. [T] People who are overweight are more likely to develop osteoarthritis than those who are not.
7. [F] Heberden nodes can occur on the middle joints of fingers.
8. [F] The ankles are a common site affected by osteoarthritis.

9. [T] With hip osteoarthritis, patients may feel pain in the knees sometimes.
10. [T] Osteoarthritis of the spine can result in numbness or weakness of the limbs.

Ⅱ. Here is a list of terms from the text. Analyze their meanings using the word building knowledge you have learned. Leave the space empty if the word part does not apply.

Term	Prefix	Combining Form /Root	Suffix	Chinese Translation
1. osteoarthritis		oste/o arthr/o	-itis	骨关节炎
2. malformation	mal-	form	-ation	畸形
3. symmetrical	sym-	metric	-al	对称的
4. degenerative	de-	generate	-ive	退化的
5. bony		bone	-y	骨的
6. osteophyte		oste/o	-phyte	骨赘
7. synovial		synovi/o	-al	滑液的

Chapter Five Digestive System

 Section A Medical Terminology

Learn the following combining forms, prefixes and suffixes for the digestive system and write the meanings of the medical terms in the space provided.

Word Part	Meaning	Example Term	Meaning in English and Chinese
amyl/o	starch 淀粉	amyloid /'æmɪlɔɪd/	resembling starch 淀粉样的
		amylolysis /ˌəmɪ'lɒlɪsɪs/	breaking down of starch 淀粉分解
an/o	anus 肛门	anoplasty /ˌænɒ'plæstɪ/	surgical repair of the anus 肛门成形术
		perianal /ˌperɪ'eɪnəl/	surrounding the anus 肛周的
append/o, appendic/o	appendix 阑尾	appendotome /ə'pendəˌtəʊm/	an instrument to cut the appendix 阑尾刀
		appendectomy /ˌəpen'dektəmɪ/	removal of the appendix 阑尾切除术
		appendicocele /ə'pendɪˌkəʊsiːl/	protrusion of the appendix 阑尾疝
		appendicitis /əˌpendə'saɪtɪs/	inflammation of the appendix 阑尾炎
-ase	enzyme 酶	lipase /'laɪpeɪz/ (*lip/o* fat)	enzyme to digest fat 脂肪酶
		amylase /'æmɪleɪz/	enzyme to digest starch 淀粉酶
cec/o	cecum 盲肠	cecorrhaphy /sɪ'kɒrəfɪ/	suture of the cecum 盲肠缝合术
		cecotomy /siː'kɒtəmɪ/	incision into the cecum 盲肠切开术
chol/e, bil/i	gall 胆 bile 胆汁	cholestasis /ˌkɒlə'stɑːsɪs/ (*-stasis* halting, stopping)	halting of the flow of bile 胆汁淤积
		cholecyst /'kɒləˌsɪst/ (*cyst/o* bladder)	gallbladder 胆囊
		bilirubin /ˌbɪlɪ'ruːbɪn/ (*-rubin* red pigment)	red pigment in bile 胆红素
		biligenesis /ˌbɪlɪ'dʒenɪsɪs/ (*-genesis* formation)	formation of the bile 胆汁生成
cholecyst/o	gallbladder 胆囊	cholecystectomy /ˌkɒlɪsɪs'tektəmɪ/	removal of the gallbladder 胆囊切除术
		cholecystitis /ˌkɒlɪsɪs'taɪtɪs/	inflammation of the gallbladder 胆囊炎

Continue

Word Part	Meaning	Example Term	Meaning in English and Chinese
col/o, colon/o	colon 结肠	colonitis /ˌkɒlə'naɪtɪs/	inflammation of the colon 结肠炎
		colopathy /kə'lɒpəθɪ/	disease of the colon 结肠病
		colonoscope /kə'lɒnəskəʊp/	an instrument to view the colon 结肠镜
		colonalgia /ˌkələʊ'nældʒɪə/	pain of the colon 结肠痛
duoden/o	duodenum 十二指肠	duodenogram /djuːə'dɪnəgræm/	X-ray record of the duodenum 十二指肠造影片
		duodenectomy /ˌdjuːədɪ'nektəmɪ/	removal of the duodenum 十二指肠切除术
gloss/o, lingu/o	tongue 舌头	glossoplasty /ˌglɒsə'plɑːstɪ/	surgical repair of the tongue 舌成形术
		glossodynia /'glɒsɒˌdɪnɪə/	pain of the tongue 舌痛
		dentolingual /ˌdentə'lɪŋgʊəl/	pertaining to teeth and tongue 齿舌(音)的
		sublingual /sʌb'lɪŋgʊəl/	under the tongue 舌下的
ile/o	ileum 回肠	ileocecal /ˌɪlɪəʊ'siːkəl/	pertaining to the ileum and cecum 回肠盲肠的
		ileorectal /ˌɪlɪəʊ'rektəl/ (*rect/o* rectum)	pertaining to the ileum and rectum 回肠直肠的
lith/o, -lith	stone 结石	lithotripsy /ˌlɪθəʊ'trɪpsɪ/ (*-tripsy* crushing)	crushing of stone 碎石术
		litholysis /lɪ'θɒləsɪs/	breaking down of stone 结石溶解
		cholelith /'kɒləlɪθ/	gall stone 胆结石
		microlith /'maɪkrəʊˌlɪθ/	small stone 小结石
-lithiasis	formation of stone 结石病	nephrolithiasis /ˌnefrəʊlɪ'θaɪəsɪs/	formation of stone in the kidney 肾结石
		cholelithiasis /ˌkɒləlɪ'θaɪəsɪs/	formation of gall stone 胆石症
-megaly	enlargement 增大	gastromegaly /ˌgəstrɒ'megəlɪ/	enlargement of the stomach 胃肥大
		enteromegaly /ˌentərəʊ'megəlɪ/	enlargement of the small intestine 肠膨大
or/o, stomat/o	mouth 口	circumoral /ˌsɜːkəm'ɔːrəl/ (*circum-* around)	around the mouth 口周的
		intra-oral /ˌɪntrə'ɔːrəl/	inside the mouth 口内的
		stomatitis /ˌstəʊmə'taɪtɪs/	inflammation of the mouth 口炎
		stomatology /ˌstəʊmə'tɒlədʒɪ/	study of the mouth 口腔学
pancreat/o	pancreas 胰腺	pancreatolith /ˌpæŋkrɪ'ætəlɪθ/	stone in the pancreas 胰石
		pancreatitis /ˌpænkrɪə'taɪtɪs/	inflammation of the pancreas 胰腺炎
-pepsia	digestion 消化	eupepsia /juː'pepsɪə/ (*eu-* good, normal)	normal digestion 消化正常
		dyspepsia /dɪs'pepsɪə/	difficulty in digestion 消化不良

Continue

Word Part	Meaning	Example Term	Meaning in English and Chinese
-pexy	surgical fixation 固定术	cecopexy /ˌsiːkə'peksɪ/	surgical fixation of the cecum 盲肠固定术
		colonopexy /ˌkəlɒnəʊ'peksɪ/	surgical fixation of the colon 结肠固定术
-phagia	eating 吃；swallowing 吞咽	polyphagia /ˌpɒlɪ'feɪdʒɪə/ (*poly-* many)	excessive eating 多食
		dysphagia /dɪs'feɪdʒɪə/	difficult in swallowing 吞咽困难
pharyng/o	pharynx 咽	pharyngitis /ˌfærɪn'dʒaɪtɪs/	inflammation of the pharynx 咽炎
		pharyngoglossal /ˌfærɪŋgəʊ'glɒsəl/	pertaining to the pharynx and tongue 咽舌的
proct/o	rectum and anus 直肠肛门，肛肠	proctoptosis /ˌprɒktɒp'təʊsɪs/ (*-ptosis* falling, sagging)	falling of the rectum outside the anus 脱肛
		proctalgia /prɒk'tældʒɪə/	pain of the rectum and anus 肛肠疼痛
splen/o	spleen 脾	splenomegaly /ˌsplenəʊ'megəlɪ/	enlargement of the spleen 脾大
		splenomalacia /ˌsplenəʊ'məleɪʃɪə/	softening of the spleen 脾软化
-stomy	surgical opening 造口术 anastomosis 吻合术	gastrostomy /gæs'trɒstəmɪ/	surgical opening from the stomach to the outside 胃造口术
		gastroduodenostomy /'gæstrəʊˌjuːdə'nɒstəmɪ/	anastomosis between the stomach and the duodenum 胃十二指肠吻合术

Exercises

Ⅰ. Fill in the following blanks with the terms in the box.

splenorrhaphy	proctologist
dyspepsia	cholelithiasis
gastrectomy	osteoblast
cholecystectomy	splenorrhexis

1. A gastrectomy is a medical procedure where all or part of the stomach is surgically removed.
2. In the car accident, Helen sustained a ruptured spleen, a condition called splenorrhexis. She was sent to a hospital and received surgical treatment, splenorrhaphy, to stitch up her spleen.
3. When you have colorectal health problems, you go to see a proctologist for thorough examination.
4. Patients suffering from stroke may have impaired swallowing function, a condition known as dysphagia, which can lead to malnutrition.
5. Indigestion, also known as dyspepsia, is a common condition marked by discomfort or pain in the stomach region.

6. Cholelithiasis is a condition in which small stones form in the gallbladder. In some patients, it can develop to intense pain as well as infection. The most typical treatment is cholecystectomy, in which the gallbladder is removed, along with the stones.

Ⅱ. Write the English and Chinese meanings of the following terms.

1. phagocyte — a swallowing cell 吞噬细胞
2. laryngospasm — involuntary contraction of the larynx 喉痉挛
3. enterocolitis — inflammation of the small intestine and colon 小肠结肠炎
4. oronasal — pertaining to the mouth and nose 口鼻的
5. glossopharyngeal — pertaining to the tongue and pharynx 舌咽的
6. amylogenic — producing starch 生成淀粉的
7. splenomegaly — enlargement of the spleen 脾大
8. colostomy — surgical opening from the colon to the outside 结肠造口术
9. enteropexy — surgical fixation of the small intestine 肠固定术
10. pancreatolithiasis — formation of stones in the pancreas 胰石病

Ⅲ. Match each word part in Column A with its English term in Column B. Write the corresponding letter in the blank provided.

	Column A	Column B
B	1. chol/e, bil/i	A. stone
D	2. -megaly	B. bile
A	3. lith/o	C. pharynx
J	4. pancreat/o	D. enlargement
E	5. or/o, stomat/o	E. mouth
I	6. -pepsia	F. swallowing
F	7. -phagia	G. enzyme
H	8. proct/o	H. rectum and anus
G	9. -ase	I. digestion
C	10. pharyng/o	J. pancreas

Section B Reading Passages

Passage One The Digestive System

Exercises

Ⅰ. Explain the meanings of the following terms in your own words.

1. mouth — The opening in the lower part of the human face, surrounded by lips, through which food is taken in, and from which speech and sounds are emitted.
2. pharynx — An organ found in humans and animals is part of the digestive system and also the respiratory system.

3. esophagus The passage, also known as foodpipe, starts from the pharynx and extends to the stomach.
4. liver An organ in your body that produces bile and cleans the blood.
5. stomach The organ inside your body where food begins to be digested.
6. gallbladder A membranous muscular sac in which bile from the liver is stored.

Ⅱ. Fill in each blank with one proper word.

Food passes down the (1) pharynx through a muscular tube called the (2) esophagus, and into a big container called the stomach, where food continues to be broken down. After its trip down the stomach, the partially digested food passes into a short tube called the (3) duodenum. The jejunum and the (4) ileum are also parts of the small intestine. Meanwhile, the accessory organs, the liver, (5) gallbladder and (6) pancreas produce enzymes and substances that help with digestion. The large intestine is where the remaining chyme goes after the nutrients have been removed. It includes the (7) cecum, colon, and (8) rectum. The (9) appendix is a branch off the large intestine, which has no known function. Now water is removed from this undigested material. The remaining product is called (10) feces and eliminated through the rectum and anus.

Ⅲ. Translate the following into English.

1. 牙周组织 periodontium
2. 会厌 epiglottis
3. 唾液腺 salivary gland
4. 十二指肠 duodenum
5. 口腔 buccal/oral cavity
6. 乙状结肠 sigmoid colon
7. 升结肠 ascending colon
8. 幽门括约肌 pyloric sphincter
9. 贲门括约肌 cardiac sphincter
10. 舌下腺 sublingual gland
11. 乳化作用 emulsification
12. 蠕动 peristalsis
13. 消化道 alimentary tract, gut
14. 下颌下腺 submandibular gland
15. 脾曲 splenic flexure

Ⅳ. Discuss the following topics.

1. What are the primary functions of the digestive system?

   The primary functions of the digestive system are as follows: ingestion—the entry of food into the body; digestion—the physical and chemical breakdown of food into nutrients that can be used by the body's cells; absorption—the passage of these nutrients from the gastrointestinal tract into the bloodstream; and elimination—the excretion of solid waste materials that cannot be absorbed into the blood.

2. Imagine you were lecturing in front of rural health workers on the topic of the digestive system, use your own word to describe the whole system.

   The answer is open.

3. Give a brief description of the functions of major organs of the digestive system.

   The oral cavity is responsible for the intake of food. The teeth are used to cut, tear, and crush food into smaller pieces. The tongue manipulates food in the mouth during mastication and deglutition. Muscles in the wall of the esophagus make rhythmic contractions that propel food. The small intestine is where nearly all of the chemical digestion of the nutritional components of food takes place. The liver produces a greenish fluid called bile which can break apart large fat globules so that enzymes from the pancreas can digest the fats. The pancreas manufactures digestive juice containing enzymes that aid in the digestion of proteins, starches and fats.

Passage Two Disorders of the Digestive System

Exercises

Ⅰ. Match each term in Column A with its correct description in Column B. Write the corresponding letter in the blank provided.

	Column A	Column B
C	1. cirrhosis	A. a substance containing bacteria that forms on the surface of the teeth
A	2. plaque	B. a protrusion of the stomach through the opening (hiatus) into the chest
G	3. appendicitis	C. chronic liver disease with degeneration of scarred liver tissue
F	4. peptic ulcer	D. inflammation of the lining of the stomach
J	5. gingivitis	E. inflammation of the pancreas
I	6. diverticulum	F. a sore or lesion of mucous membrane of the stomach caused by the action of peptic juice
B	7. hiatal hernia	G. an illness in which the appendix is infected and painful
E	8. pancreatitis	H. a substance added to another to make it less hard
D	9. gastritis	I. any sac or pouch by herniation of the wall of a tubular（管状的）organ or part, especially the intestines
H	10. softener	J. a gum disease caused by bacterial plaque

Ⅱ. Fill in each blank with a correct term in the box. Change the form of the words if necessary.

small intestine	hepatitis	gallstone	cholecystectomy	
cirrhosis	appendicitis	colon	diaphragm	diverticulosis

1. Hepatitis is a medical condition defined by the inflammation of the liver and characterized by the presence of inflammatory cells in the tissue of the organ.
2. In the United States the most common causes of acute pancreatitis are gallstones and heavy alcohol use.
3. Low-fiber diets in developed or industrial countries may lead to diverticulosis.
4. Peptic ulcer disease is a break in the lining of the stomach, first part of the small intestine, or occasionally the lower esophagus.
5. Cirrhosis is often preceded by hepatitis and fatty liver, independent of the cause.

6. A hiatal hernia is the protrusion of the upper part of the stomach into the thorax through a tear or weakness in the diaphragm.
7. Cholecystectomy, performed via an abdominal incision below the lower right ribs, has a 99% chance of eliminating the recurrence of cholelithiasis.
8. Abdominal pain, nausea, vomiting, and lasting fever are considered as the classic presentations of acute appendicitis.
9. Colorectal cancer is the development of cancer in the colon or rectum.

Ⅲ. Translate the following sentences into Chinese.

1. The ultimate danger of chronic liver disease is the development of cirrhosis with its complications and liver cancer.
   慢性肝病中最严重的是肝硬化导致的并发症和肝癌。
2. Peptic ulcers can be diagnosed by endoscopy and by X-ray studies of the upper gastrointestinal tract using a contrast medium, usually barium.
   消化溃疡可通过内镜检查来诊断，也可用造影剂（通常为钡）对胃肠道上段进行 X 线检查来诊断。
3. H. pylori is a bacterial infection of the stomach that does not cause any problem until a person develops ulcers.
   幽门螺杆菌感染是胃部的一种细菌性感染，胃溃疡发病前，它不会引起任何麻烦。
4. Drugs may be used to dissolve gallstones, but often the cure is removal of the gallbladder.
   胆结石可用药物溶解，但治愈常常是要依靠切除胆囊。
5. Ulcerative colitis encompasses a spectrum of diffuse, continuous, superficial inflammation of the colon that begins within the rectum and extends to a variable level.
   溃疡性结肠炎包括一系列扩散、持续和浅表的结肠炎症。它起自直肠，发展至不同的部位。

Ⅳ. Discuss the following topics.

1. What are the causes of digestive diseases?
   The causes of many digestive diseases remain unknown. They may be inherited or develop from multiple factors such as stress, fatigue, diet, or smoking. Abusing alcohol imposes the greatest risk for digestive diseases.
2. What are the known types of hepatitis virus?
   There are several known types of hepatitis virus, but the main ones are hepatitis A virus (HAV) and hepatitis B virus (HBV). Type A is spread by fecal-oral contamination, often by food handlers and in crowded, unsanitary conditions. Type B is caused by blood and blood products, and may also be transmitted sexually. Individuals may become carriers of the disease. Most cases of hepatitis following transfusion are now caused by type C.
3. What are the causes of colorectal cancer?
   A diet low in fiber and calcium and high in fat is a major risk factor for colorectal cancer. Heredity is also a factor, as is chronic inflammation of the colon.

Passage Three Peptic Ulcer

Exercises

Ⅰ. Read the following statements and decide whether they are true or false. Then write T for true and F for false in the brackets.

1. [F] Most people who have ulcers have belly pain or other symptoms.
2. [F] NSAIDs are typically used to treat peptic ulcers.
3. [F] Eating a good meal can usually make ulcer patients who have abdominal pain feel better.
4. [F] Bleeding from an ulcer usually means a medical emergency.
5. [T] EGD can detect small ulcers and treat bleeding directly.
6. [F] PPIs should be taken before meals or one hour after meals.
7. [F] A blood test will usually tell us whether the H. pylori infection is gone.
8. [T] People with ulcers should stop taking NSAIDs if possible.
9. [F] Depression is an important cause of ulcers.
10. [F] People with an ulcer should follow a specific diet and avoid spicy foods.

Ⅱ. Fill in each blank with a correct term in the box. Change the form of the words if necessary.

complication	abdominal	gastric	H. pylori
duodenal	symptom	NSAID	intestinal

Peptic ulcer disease (PUD), also known as a peptic ulcer or stomach ulcer, is a break in the lining of the stomach, first part of the small intestine, or occasionally the lower esophagus. An ulcer in the stomach is known as a (1) gastric ulcer while that in the first part of the intestines is known as a (2) duodenal ulcer. The most common symptoms are waking at night with upper (3) abdominal pain. Other symptoms include belching, vomiting, weight loss, or poor appetite. About a third of older people have no symptoms. (4) Complications may include bleeding, perforation, and blockage of the stomach. Common causes include infection of the stomach by bacteria called (5) H. pylori and the use of (6) NSAIDs, which include aspirin, ibuprofen, and naproxen. Other less common causes include tobacco smoking and drinking too much alcohol.

Chapter Six Respiratory System

Section A Medical Terminology

Learn the following combining forms, prefixes and suffixes for the respiratory system and write the meanings of the medical terms in the space provided.

Word Part	Meaning	Example Term	Meaning in English and Chinese
bronch/o, bronchi/o	bronchus, bronchial tube 支气管	bronchogenic /ˌbrɒnkə'dʒenɪk/ (*-genic* originated from)	originated from the bronchus 支气管原的
		bronchitis /brɒŋ'kaɪtɪs/	inflammation of the bronchus 支气管炎
		peribronchial /ˌperɪ'brɒnkɪəl/	surrounding the bronchus 支气管周的
		bronchiospasm /'brɒŋkɪəʊˌspæzəm/	involuntary contraction of the bronchus 支气管痉挛
-capnia	level of carbon dioxide (in blood) 二氧化碳（血）量	eucapnia /juː'kæpnɪə/ (*eu-* good, normal)	normal carbon dioxide level (in blood) 血碳正常
		hypercapnia /ˌhaɪpə'kæpnɪə/	high carbon dioxide level (in blood) 高碳酸血症
cyan/o	blue 青，发绀	acrocyanosis /ˌækrəʊsaɪə'nəʊsɪs/	bluish discoloration of the extremities 肢端发绀
		cyanotic /saɪə'nɒtɪk/	pertaining to bluish discoloration of the skin 发绀的
-ectasia, -ectasis	dilation 扩张	atelectasis /ˌætə'lektəsɪs/ (*atel/o* incomplete)	incomplete dilation (of the lung) 肺不张
		bronchiectasia /ˌbrɒŋkɪ'ektəsɪə /	dilation of the bronchus 气管扩张
epiglott/o	epiglottis 会厌	hypoepiglottic /ˌhaɪpəʊˌepɪ'glɒtɪk/	below the epiglottis 会厌下的
		epiglottoplasty /ˌepɪˌglɒtəʊ'plæstɪ/	surgical repair of the epiglottis 会厌软骨成形术
laryng/o	larynx 喉	laryngocentesis /ˌlərɪŋˌgəʊsen'tiːsɪs/	surgical puncture into the larynx 喉穿刺术
		laryngostomy /ˌlærɪŋ'gɒstəmɪ/	surgical opening from the larynx to the outside 喉造口术

Continue

Word Part	Meaning	Example Term	Meaning in English and Chinese
lob/o	lobe, leaf 叶	lobule /'lɒbjuːl/ (*-ule* small thing)	a small lobe 小叶
		lobectomy /ləʊ'bektəmɪ/	removal of a lobe（肺）叶切除术
medi-	middle 中间	mediastinum /ˌmiːdɪæ'staɪnəm/	the space between the two lungs 正中隔，纵隔
		median /'miːdɪən/	pertaining to the middle 正中的，中央的
-oxia	level of oxygen 氧量	hypoxia /haɪ'pɒksɪə/	low level of oxygen 缺氧
		anoxia /æ'nɒksɪə/	without oxygen 无氧；缺氧
ox/i	oxygen 氧	oxidase /'ɒksɪdeɪs/	enzyme to catalyze biological oxidation 氧化酶
		oximeter /ɒk'sɪmɪtə/	an instrument to measure oxygen (in blood) 血氧计
pleur/o	pleura 胸膜	pleurodynia /ˌplʊərəʊ'dɪnɪə/	pain of the pleura 胸膜痛
		pleurocentesis /ˌplʊərəsen'tiːsɪs/	surgical puncture into the pleural cavity 胸膜穿刺术
-pnea	breathing 呼吸	dyspnea /dɪs'pniːə/	difficult, painful breathing 呼吸困难
		eupnea /juː'pniːə/	normal breathing 呼吸正常
pneum/o, pneumon/o	air 空气；lung 肺	pneumothorax /ˌnjuːmə'θɔːræks/	presence of air in the chest 气胸
		pneumocardial /ˌnjuːmə'kaːdɪəl/	pertaining to the lung and heart 肺心的
		pneumatosis /ˌnjuːmə'təʊsɪs/	abnormal accumulation of air 积气
		pneumatometry /ˌnjuːmə'tɔːmɪtrɪ/	process of measuring the volume of breathing 呼吸气量测定法
-ptysis	spitting 咯，咳	hemoptysis /hɪ'mɒptəsɪs/	spitting of blood 咯血
		blennoptysis /ble'nɒptəsɪs/ (*blenn/o* mucus)	spitting of mucus 黏液痰
pulmon/o	lung 肺	intrapulmonary /ˌɪntrə'pʌlməˌnərɪ/	within the lungs 肺内的
		pulmonary /'pʌlməˌnərɪ/	pertaining to the lung 肺的
py/o	pus 脓	pyoptysis /paɪ'ɒptəsɪs/	spitting of pus 咯脓
		pyogenesis /ˌpaɪə'dʒenəsɪs/	formation of pus 化脓
-stenosis	narrowing 狭窄	bronchostenosis /ˌbrɒnkəʊstɪ'nəʊsɪs/	narrowing of the bronchus 支气管狭窄
		laryngostenosis /ləˌrɪŋgəʊstɪ'nəʊsɪs/	narrowing of the larynx 喉狭窄
trache/o	trachea 气管	tracheorrhaphy /træ'kɔːrəfɪ/	surgical suture of the trachea 气管缝合术
		tracheostomy /ˌtrækɪ'ɒstəmɪ/	surgical opening from the trachea to the outside 气管造口术

Exercises

Ⅰ. Fill in the following blanks with the terms in the box.

cyanosis	bronchoplasty
bronchostenosis	tracheostomy
bronchogenic	hypoxia
dyspnea	pneumothorax
lobectomy	hemoptysis

1. A tracheostomy is a surgical procedure to create an opening through the neck into the trachea (windpipe) to bypass an obstructed upper airway.
2. When the bronchus is narrowed, a condition known as bronchostenosis, the flow of air in and out of the lung is restricted. This can be a chronic condition when there is accumulation of scar tissue on the bronchus, which can be treated with bronchoplasty, to surgically repair the structure of a bronchus.
3. Coughing up blood, or hemoptysis, is one of the important symptoms of cardiopulmonary disease because bleeding even in small amounts may indicate the presence of serious diseases like cancer or tuberculosis.
4. A collapsed lung is a build-up of air in the space between the lung and the pleural cavity. This condition is also known as pneumothorax. Patients will show bluish discoloration of the skin, or cyanosis, as a result of lacking oxygen supply, hypoxia.
5. With conditions concerning the respiratory system, difficulty in breathing, or dyspnea, is often experienced.
6. A lobectomy is a type of lung cancer surgery in which one lobe of a lung is removed. If the cancer originates from the bronchus, it is called a bronchogenic lung cancer.

Ⅱ. Write the English and Chinese meanings of the following terms.

1. pharyngolaryngeal pertaining to the pharynx and the larynx 咽喉的
2. tracheobronchitis inflammation of the trachea and the bronchus 气管支气管炎
3. laryngoscope an instrument to examine the larynx 喉镜
4. hyperoxia high level of oxygen (in blood) 高氧症
5. apnea without breathing, cessation of breathing 无呼吸；呼吸暂停
6. pyothorax presence of pus in the chest 脓胸
7. pharyngostenosis narrowing of the pharynx 咽狭窄
8. tracheoscopy examination of the trachea using an endoscope 气管镜检查
9. pneumectomy excision of the lung 肺切除术
10. bronchiectasia dilation of the bronchus 支气管扩张

Ⅲ. Match each word part in Column A with its English term in Column B. Write the corresponding letter in the blank provided.

Column A	Column B
D 1. -oxia	A. pleura

Answer	Term		Meaning
J	2. -ectasia, -ectasis		B. air, lung
H	3. lob/o		C. pus
A	4. pleur/o		D. oxygen level
B	5. pneum/o, pneumon/o		E. trachea
I	6. -capnia		F. narrowing
G	7. cyan/o		G. blue
C	8. py/o		H. lobe, leaf
E	9. trache/o		I. carbon dioxide level
F	10. -stenosis		J. dilation

Section B Reading Passages

Passage One Respiratory System

Exercises

Ⅰ. Explain the meanings of the following terms in your own words.

1. oral cavity — The opening through which many animals take in food and issue vocal sounds.
2. trachea — A tube, colloquially called windpipe, connects the pharynx and larynx to the lungs, and allows the passage of air.
3. larynx — An organ which is commonly called the voice box in the neck of humans and involved in breathing, sound production, and protecting the trachea against food aspiration.
4. lung — One of the two organs in your body that you breathe with.
5. heart — The organ in your chest which pumps blood through your body.
6. ribs — The 12 pairs of curved bones that surround your chest.

Ⅱ. Fill in each blank with one proper word or phrase.

The lungs are two cone-shaped, spongy organs consisting of alveoli, blood vessels, elastic tissue and nerves. Each of the two lungs consists of smaller divisions called (1) lobes. The left lung has two lobes while the right lung is divided into three lobes. In the lungs, (2) alveoli are surrounded by a network of tiny blood vessels called capillaries; (3) oxygen from the lungs passes into these capillaries for distribution to tissue cells, while carbon dioxide from the blood passes into the lungs to be expelled by (4) exhalation. Once absorbed into blood cells, oxygen becomes attached to (5) hemoglobin and is released to tissue cells as needed. Thus, the primary function of the lungs is to bring air into close contact with blood, which allows (6) gas exchange to occur.

The lungs are surrounded by a membrane called the (7) visceral pleura. The space that the lungs occupy within the chest is called the (8) thoracic cavity, which is lined by a membrane called the parietal pleura. The parietal and visceral pleurae lie very close to each other; the small space between these membranes, called the (9) pleural space, is filled with a fluid that prevents friction when the two membranes slide against each other during respiration. A group of smooth muscles called the (10) diaphragm separates the lower portion of the thoracic cavity from the abdomen.

Ⅲ. Translate the following into English.

1. 鼻旁窦	paranasal sinus	2. 滞痰	stagnant sputum
3. 口咽	oropharynx	4. 食管	esophagus
5. 呼出	expiration/exhalation	6. 纵隔	mediastinum
7. 肺泡	alveolus	8. 扁桃体	tonsils
9. 二氧化碳	carbon dioxide	10. 酸中毒	acidosis
11. 肺换气不足	hypoventilation	12. 胸膜	visceral pleura
13. 咽喉	laryngopharynx	14. 污染物	pollutant

Ⅳ. Discuss the following topics.

1. Imagine you were lecturing in front of rural health workers on the topic of the respiratory system, use your own words to describe the whole system.
   The respiratory system is involved in the intake and exchange of oxygen and carbon dioxide between an organism and the environment. The major organs of the respiratory system are the nose, pharynx, larynx, trachea, bronchi and lungs.
2. How can epiglottis prevent the passing food and drink from entering the respiratory system?
   The epiglottis lies over the entrance to the larynx. In the act of swallowing, when food and liquid move through the throat, the epiglottis closes off the larynx so that these things cannot enter.
3. What role does the diaphragm play in the process of breathing?
   The diaphragm aids in the process of breathing. It contracts and descends with each inhalation. The downward movement of the diaphragm enlarges the area in the thoracic cavity and reduces the internal air pressure, so that air flows into the lungs to equalize the pressure. When the lungs are full, the diaphragm relaxes and elevates, making the area in the thoracic cavity smaller and thus increasing the air pressure in the thorax. Air is then expelled out of the lungs to equalize the pressure, which is called exhalation.

Passage Two Respiratory Disorders and Diseases

Exercises

Ⅰ. Match each term in Column A with its correct description in Column B. Write the corresponding letter in the blank provided.

Column A	Column B
__D__ 1. dyspnea	A. the spitting or couching up of blood
__C__ 2. bronchiectasis	B. chronic respiratory disease caused by inhaling metallic or mineral particles

Answer	Term	Definition
F	3. hypoxia	C. chronic enlargement of bronchial tubes
B	4. pneumoconiosis	D. difficulty in breathing
J	5. asthma	E. inflammation of the bronchi persisting for a long time
I	6. emphysema	F. lack of oxygen in the tissue
E	7. chronic bronchitis	G. one form of pneumoconiosis arising from inhalation of coal and quartz dust
H	8. tuberculosis	H. infection transmitted by inhalation or ingestion of tubercle bacilli and manifested in fever and small lesions
G	9. anthracosilicosis	I. a chronic lung disease associated with overexpansion and destruction of the alveoli
A	10. hemoptysis	J. bronchial airway obstruction due to spasm of bronchi

Ⅱ. Fill in each blank with a correct term in the box. Change the form of the words if necessary.

pulmonary edema	alveolus	wheeze	fever	pneumothorax
pneumoconiosis	pleura	emphysema	silicosis	influenza virus

1. A pneumothorax is an abnormal collection of air or gas in the pleural space that causes an uncoupling of the lung from the chest wall.
2. Influenza, commonly known as “the flu”, is an infectious disease caused by an influenza virus.
3. Pneumonia is an inflammatory condition of the lung affecting primarily the microscopic air sacs known as alveoli.
4. Pleurisy (also known as pleuritis) is an inflammation of the pleura, the lining surrounding the lungs.
5. Pneumoconiosis is an occupational and a restrictive lung disease caused by the inhalation of dust, often in mines.
6. Asthma is characterized by recurrent episodes of wheezing, shortness of breath, chest tightness, and coughing.
7. Long-term exposure to the irritants causes an inflammatory response in the lungs resulting in narrowing of the small airways and breakdown of lung tissue, known as emphysema.
8. Silicosis is a form of occupational lung disease caused by inhalation of crystalline silica dust.
9. General signs and symptoms of tuberculosis include fever, weight loss, weakness, cough and fatigue.
10. Pulmonary edema is an abnormal buildup of fluid in the lungs. This buildup of fluid leads to shortness of breath.

Ⅲ. Translate the following sentences into Chinese.

1. Pleurisy is severe chest pain accompanying each deep breath in a person with an inflamed pleura, the twin membrane surrounding each lung and lining the chest cavity.
   胸膜炎是指包绕每个肺叶和胸腔内层的双层膜，即胸膜发炎，深呼吸时，病人会有剧烈的胸疼。

2. Tuberculosis has increased in recent years along with the rise of AIDS and the appearance of resistance to antibiotics in the organism that causes the disease.
   近年来，随着艾滋病发病率的上升以及出现致病微生物对抗生素抗药性，肺结核的发病率也在攀升。
3. Although the cause of asthma is uncertain, foreign particles such as pollen or certain environmental pollutants are believed to be the culprits, which stimulate the smooth muscle of the bronchial tree to release histamine causing the muscle to contract.
   虽然哮喘的病因尚不清楚，但一些异物如花粉和某些环境污染物被认为是主要元凶，它们刺激支气管树平滑肌，使之释放出组织胺，造成肌肉收缩。
4. The fluid buildup is caused by heart trouble that, in turn, produces back pressure in the pulmonary veins and the left atrium of the heart to which they carry oxygen-rich blood from the lungs.
   由心脏病引起的体液积累会对肺静脉和左心房产生反压，影响富氧血从肺部输出，进而导致血氧含量降低而发绀。
5. Emphysema, another lung response to noxious stimuli, is characterized by abnormal, permanent enlargement of air spaces distal to the terminal bronchioles, accompanied by destruction of their walls, and without obvious fibrosis.
   肺气肿是肺对有害刺激的另一种反应，即末端细支气管远侧气道的异常、持续性增大，伴随其壁受损但没有明显的纤维变性。

Ⅳ. Discuss the following topics.

1. Name three respiratory diseases mentioned in this passage, list their symptoms and signs and then explain the possible causative factors.
   Pleurisy is severe chest pain accompanying each deep breath in a person with an inflamed pleura, the twin membrane surrounding each lung and lining the chest cavity. Pleurisy can attend pneumonia or result from direct infection of the pleura.
   Pneumothorax occurs when air gets into the chest between the pleural lining. The lung then cannot fully expand and breathing becomes difficult. As a result, the lung may even collapse. Pneumothorax may result from a wound in the chest, such as a knife wound, or after a sudden tear in the lung. Infection of the pleural space by gas-producing microbes can also cause pneumothorax.
   Acute pulmonary edema results when fluid quickly accumulates in the lungs and fills the alveoli. The fluid buildup is caused by heart trouble that, in turn, produces back pressure in the pulmonary veins and the left atrium of the heart to which they carry oxygen-rich blood from the lungs. A person suffering acute pulmonary edema is suddenly breathless and turns blue because of oxygen-poor blood.
2. Which four chronic diseases are included in chronic obstructive pulmonary disease?
   The four chronic diseases are simple chronic bronchitis, chronic obstructive bronchitis, asthmatic bronchitis and emphysema.

3. Why is chronic obstructive bronchitis also called small airways disease?
   Because the obstruction is in the bronchioles and bronchi two mm or less in diameter.

Passage Three How Is Asthma Treated and Controlled?

Exercises

Ⅰ. Read the following statements and decide whether they are true or false. Then write T for true and F for false in the brackets.

1. [F] Asthma is an chronic disease that can be cured.
2. [T] Good asthma control can help you sleep better.
3. [T] Your asthma action plan should tell you what asthma triggers to avoid and how to deal with an emergency.
4. [F] All of the asthma triggers should be identified and avoided.
5. [F] Inhaled corticosteroids are the best choice when asthma attacks.
6. [T] Osteoporosis may occur as a side effect of taking corticosteroid.
7. [F] If thrush occurs, you may have to switch to another long-term asthma control medicine.
8. [T] If your child has asthma, his or her school should also be informed.
9. [F] Inhaled short-acting beta2-agonists can relax tight muscles around your airways and reduce airway inflammation.
10. [T] Asthma patients should take quick-relief medicines with them when they go traveling.

Ⅱ. Fill in each blank with a correct term in the box. Change the form of the words if necessary.

treatment	diagnosis	mental	wheeze
chronic	allergen	environmental	acute

Asthma is a common (1) chronic inflammatory disease of the airways characterized by variable and recurring symptoms, reversible airflow obstruction and bronchospasm. Common symptoms include (2) wheezing, coughing, chest tightness, and shortness of breath. Asthma is thought to be caused by a combination of genetic and (3) environmental factors. Its (4) diagnosis is usually based on the pattern of symptoms, response to therapy over time and spirometry. Treatment of (5) acute symptoms is usually with an inhaled short-acting beta2-agonists and oral corticosteroids. In very severe cases, intravenous corticosteroids, magnesium sulfate, and hospitalization may be required. Symptoms can be prevented by avoiding triggers, such as (6) allergens and irritants, and by the use of inhaled corticosteroids.

Chapter Seven Cardiovascular System

Section A Medical Terminology

Learn the following combining forms, prefixes and suffixes for the cardiovascular system and write the meanings of the medical terms in the space provided.

Word Part	Meaning	Example Term	Meaning in English and Chinese
aort/o	aorta 主动脉	aortitis /ˌeɪɔːˈtaɪtɪs/	inflammation of the aorta 主动脉炎
		aortopathy /ˌeɪɔːˈtəʊpəθɪ/	disease of the aorta 主动脉病
arteri/o	artery 动脉	arteriostenosis /ˌɑːtɪəriːəʊsteˈnəʊsɪs/	narrowing of the artery 动脉狭窄
		arterioplasty /ˌɑːtɪəriːəʊˈplæstɪ/	surgical repair of the artery 动脉修补术
atri/o	atrium 心房	interatrial /ˌɪntəˈeɪtrɪəl/	between the atria 心房间的
		atriomegaly /ˌeɪtrɪəˈmegəlɪ/	enlargement of the atrium 心房肥大
brady-	slow 慢	bradycardia /ˌbrædɪˈkɑːdɪə/	slow heart beat 心动徐缓
		bradyrhythmia /ˌbrædɪˈrɪθmɪə/	slow heart rhythm 心搏徐缓
cardi/o	heart 心	cardiopathy /ˌkɑːdɪˈɒpəθɪ/	disease of the heart 心脏病
		cardiology /ˌkɑːdɪˈɒlədʒɪ/	study of the heart 心脏病学
coron/o	crown 冠状	coronary /ˈkɒrənərɪ/	pertaining to the crown 冠的；冠状的
		coronoid /ˈkɒrənɔɪd/	resembling the crown 冠状的
-cuspid	pointed shape 尖的	tricuspid /traɪˈkʌspɪd/	having three points 三尖的；三尖瓣的
		bicuspid /baɪˈkʌspɪd/	having two points 二尖的；二尖瓣的
echo-	high-frequency sound waves 超声回波	echocardiography /ˌekəʊkɑːdɪˈɒgrəfɪ/	process of recording the heart using high-frequency waves 超声心动描记术
		echogram /ˈekəʊˌgræm/	image produced by the high-frequency wave 回声图
embol/o	mass of clotted blood 栓塞	embolism /ˈembəˌlɪzəm/	obstruction of a blood vessel by an embolus 栓塞
		emboliform /ɪmˈbəʊlɪfɔːm/	in the form of embolus 栓子状的

Continue

Word Part	Meaning	Example Term	Meaning in English and Chinese
-genic	produced by or producing 产生	cardiogenic /ˌkɑːdɪəʊ'dʒenɪk/	resulting from the heart 心源性的
		pathogenic /ˌpæθə'dʒenɪk/	producing the disease 致病的
isch-	hold back, suppress 闭；缺	ischemia /ɪs'kiːmɪə/	reduced blood supply 缺血
		ischocholia /ˌɪskəʊ'kəʊlɪə/(*chol/e* bile)	suppression of bile secretion 胆汁抑制
-ole	little, small 小	arteriole /ɑː'tɪərɪəʊl/	small branch of an artery 小动脉
		bronchiole /'brɒŋkɪəʊl/	small bronchial tube 细支气管
phleb/o, ven/o	vein 静脉	phlebitis /flə'baɪtɪs/	inflammation of the vein 静脉炎
		phleboplasty /ˌfləbəʊ'plæstɪ/	surgical repair of the vein 静脉成形术
		intravenous /ˌɪntrə'viːnəs/	inside the vein 静脉内的
		arteriovenous /ˌɑːtɪəriːəʊ'viːnəs /	pertaining to arteries and veins 动静脉的
semi-	half 半 partial 部分	semilunar /ˌsemɪ'luːnə/ (*-lunar* the moon)	shaped like half a moon 半月状的
		semipermeable /ˌsemɪ'pɜːmɪəbl/	partially permeable 半渗透的
-sclerosis	hardening 硬化	atherosclerosis/ˌæθərəʊsklɪ'rəʊsɪs/ (*ather/o* plaque of fatty substance)	hardening of the artery due to deposit of fatty substance 动脉粥样硬化
		arterioscleros is /ˌɑːtərəʊsklɪ'rəʊsɪs/	hardening of the artery 动脉硬化
sphygm/o	pulse 脉	sphygmomanometer/ˌsfɪgməʊmə'nɒmɪtə/ (*mano-* pressure)	instrument to measure the pressure of the pulse 血压计
		sphygmoscopy /'sfɪgməʊˌskəpɪ/	examination of the pulse 脉搏检查
tachy-	fast 快	tachycardia /ˌtækɪ'kɑːdɪə/	fast heart beat 心动过速
		tachypnea /ˌtækɪp'niːə/ (*-pnea* breathing)	fast breathing 呼吸过速
thromb/o	clot 血栓	thrombosis /θrɒm'bəʊsɪs/	formation of a thrombus 血栓形成
		thrombophlebitis/ˌθrɒmbəʊflɪ'baɪtɪs/	inflammation of a vein due to thrombus 血栓性静脉炎
valvul/o	valve 瓣膜	valvuloplasty /'vælvjʊləˌplæstɪ/	surgical repair of the valve 瓣膜成形术
		valvulitis /ˌvælvjʊ'laɪtɪs/	inflammation of the valve 瓣膜炎
vas/o	vessel 血管	vasoactive /ˌveɪzəʊ'æktɪv/	acting on the vessels 血管活性的
		vasopressor /ˌveɪzəʊ'presə/ (*-pressor* an agent to stimulate contraction)	an agent to stimulate the contraction of the vessel 血管加压剂
ventricul/o	ventricle of the heart or the brain 心 / 脑室	interventricular /ˌɪntəven'trɪkjʊlə/	between the ventricles 心 / 脑室间的
		ventriculotomy/ˌventrɪkjʊ'ləʊtəʊmɪ/	incision into a ventricle 心 / 脑室切开术

Exercises

I. Fill in the following blanks with the terms in the box.

cardiogenic	interventricular
aortocoronary	valvuloplasty
tachykinesis	atrioventricular
bradykinesis	thrombolytic
vasodilator	vasopressor

1. A cardiogenic shock is caused by a condition originating from the heart.
2. An interventricular septum separates the two ventricles while an atrioventricular septum separates the upper and lower heart chambers.
3. Valvuloplasty is surgical repair of a deformed cardiac valve.
4. If you know *-kinesis* means movement, then fast movement is termed tachykinesis and slow movement is called bradykinesis.
5. A vasodilator is an agent that dilates the blood vessels and a vasopressor is an agent that contracts the blood vessels.
6. A thrombolytic drug can break up or dissolve the thrombus that blocks the flow of blood.
7. A patient suffers from coronary heart disease and his doctor recommends an aortocoronary bypass surgery to shunt the blood from aorta to branches of coronary arteries to increase the supply of blood to the heart muscle.

II. Write a word for each of the following definitions.

1. pertaining to the heart and blood vessels cardiovascular
2. disease of the heart muscle cardiomyopathy
3. between the ventricles interventricular
4. inflammation of the artery arteritis
5. pertaining to the valve valvular
6. pertaining to the atrium and the ventricle atrioventricular
7. hardening of the vein phlebosclerosis/venosclerosis
8. involuntary contraction of the artery arterospasm
9. enlargement of the heart cardiomegaly
10. disease of the valve valvulopathy

III. Match each word part in Column A with its English term in Column B. Write the corresponding letter in the blank provided.

	Column A	Column B
H	1. ven/o, phleb/o	A. atrium
F	2. aort/o	B. heart
C	3. -cuspid	C. pointed

__I__ 4. vas/o D. crown
__B__ 5. cardi/o E. clot
__E__ 6. thromb/o F. aorta
__J__ 7. sphygm/o G. half, partial
__G__ 8. semi- H. vein
__D__ 9. coron/o I. vessel
__A__ 10. atri/o J. pulse

Section B Reading Passages

Passage One The Cardiovascular System

Exercises

Ⅰ. Explain the meanings of the following terms in your own words.

1. pulmonary artery An artery that carries deoxygenated blood from the heart to the lungs.
2. veins Blood vessels that carry deoxygenated blood from the tissues back to the heart, with the exceptions of the pulmonary and umbilical veins which carry oxygenated blood to the heart.
3. atrium The atrium is the upper chamber in which blood enters the heart. There are two atria in the human heart—the left atrium connected to the lungs, and the right atrium connected to the venous circulation.
4. ventricle A ventricle is one of two large chambers toward the bottom of the heart that collect and expel blood received from an atrium.
5. vena cava The venae cavae (from the Latin for "hollow veins", singular "vena cava") are large veins that return deoxygenated blood from the body into the heart. In humans they are called the superior vena cava and the inferior vena cava, and both empty into the right atrium.
6. aorta The aorta is the main artery in the human body, originating from the left ventricle of the heart and extending down to the abdomen, where it splits into two smaller arteries. The aorta distributes oxygenated blood to all parts of the body through the systemic circulation.

Ⅱ. Fill in each blank with one proper word.

Blood returning from the body tissues enters the right (1) atrium, which is the upper chamber on the right side of the (2) heart. When the muscles of this chamber contract, they force the blood into the right (3) ventricle, which is the major pump chamber on the right side of the heart. When the ventricle muscle (4) contracts, it forces blood out through the (5) pulmonary artery and through the small blood vessels of the lungs. In these small lung vessels, the blood is separated from air by very thin membranes, and oxygen (6) enters the blood and carbon dioxide

(7) leaves the blood by simple diffusion. This cleaned and refreshed (8) blood then passes into the left ventricle which is powerful, and when it contracts, it pushes the blood, under considerable pressure, into the (9) systemic circulation by means of a large artery called the (10) aorta.

Ⅲ. Translate the following into English.

1. 主动脉弓	aortic arch	2. 胸动脉	thoracic aorta
3. 舒张压	diastolic pressure	4. 腹主动脉	abdominal aorta
5. 收缩压	systolic pressure	6. 脊柱	vertebral column/spinal column/ backbone
7. 毫米汞柱	millimeter mercury (mmHg)	8. 半月形瓣	semilunar valve
9. 室间隔	interventricular septum	10. 升主动脉	ascending aorta
11. 二尖瓣	mitral valve/ bicuspid valve	12. 体循环	systemic circuit
13. 上腔静脉	superior vena cava	14. 下腔静脉	inferior vena cava
15. 心肌	myocardium	16. 心内膜	endocardium
17. 小静脉	venule	18. 心外膜	epicardium
19. 小动脉	arteriole	20. 心包	pericardium

Ⅳ. Discuss the following topics.

1. Compare pulmonary circulation and systemic circulation.

   Blood flows in two closed circuits, the pulmonary circulation and the systemic circulation. As part of the systemic circulation, oxygen-rich blood flows from the aorta (the largest blood vessel in the body) to the coronary artery to nourish the heart. In pulmonary circulation, the pulmonary arteries carry blood low in oxygen from the right ventricle while the pulmonary veins carry blood high in oxygen from the lungs into the left atrium. This circuit concerns itself with eliminating carbon dioxide from the blood and replenishing its supply of oxygen.

2. Draw a picture to illustrate the four chambers of the heart and then discuss their locations and functions.

   The answer is open.

3. Give a brief description of the blood vessels.

   There are three major types of blood vessels, i.e., arteries, veins, and capillaries. Arteries lead blood away from the heart. Veins conduct waste-filled blood toward the heart from the tissues. Capillaries have thin and transparent walls that allow passage of oxygen and nutrients out of the bloodstream and into the tissue fluid surrounding the cells. At the same time, waste products such as carbon dioxide and water pass out of the cells and into the capillaries.

Passage Two Common Disorders of the Cardiovascular System

Exercises

Ⅰ. Match each term in Column A with its correct description in Column B. Write the corresponding letter in the blank provided.

Column A	Column B
D 1. phlebitis	A. a distended or tortuous（扭曲的）vein

H	2. hemorrhage	B. inflammation of a vein with blood clotting
G	3. coronary occlusion	C. abnormally high blood pressure
F	4. endocarditis	D. inflammation of a vein
J	5. pericarditis	E. deficiency of blood flow
I	6. angina pectoris	F. inflammation of the inner lining of the heart
B	7. thrombophlebitis	G. obstruction of an artery of the heart
E	8. ischemia	H. escape of blood from vessels
A	9. varicose vein	I. chest pain due to insufficient blood supply to the heart muscle
C	10. hypertension	J. inflammation of the membrane surrounding the heart

Ⅱ. Fill in each blank with a correct term in the box. Change the form of the words if necessary.

rheumatic fever	hypertrophy	heart failure	secondary
endocarditis	essential	atherosclerosis	hemorrhoid
myocardial infarction	embolus	cardiac tamponade	

1. Elevated blood pressure of unknown cause is called essential hypertension while blood pressure which is elevated as a result of another condition is called secondary hypertension.
2. Death of a portion of myocardial muscle caused by lack of oxygen resulting from an interrupted blood supply is called myocardial infarction.
3. Rheumatic heart disease is a type of heart disease caused by rheumatic fever.
4. Varicose veins near the anus are called hemorrhoids.
5. Hardening of fatty plaque deposited on the arterial wall is called atherosclerosis.
6. Acute compression of the heart caused by fluid accumulation in the pericardial cavity is known as cardiac tamponade.
7. Heart failure is the inability of the heart to pump blood at an adequate rate to meet tissue metabolic requirements or the ability to do so only at an elevated filling pressure.
8. A blood clot or foreign material that enters the bloodstream and moves until it lodges at another point in the circulation is called an embolus.
9. Vegetation of the heart valves may occur as a result of endocarditis.
10. Enlargement of the left ventricular wall, usually occurring as a result of chronic hypertension, is called left ventricular hypertrophy.

Ⅲ. Translate the following sentences into Chinese.

1. Such bleeding may be external or internal, from vessels of any size, and may involve any part of the body.
   出血分为外出血和内出血，可来自任何大小的血管，可涉及身体的任何部位。
2. One of its symptoms is angina pectoris, which is manifested as a feeling of constriction around the heart or pain radiating to the left arm or shoulder, usually brought on by exertion.

其中一个症状是心绞痛，表现为心脏周围的压榨感或向左臂 / 左肩辐射的疼痛，常因用力而诱发。

3. Damming back of blood caused by right-sided heart failure results in accumulation of fluid in the abdominal organs (liver and spleen) and subcutaneous tissue of the legs.
   右心衰所致的血液淤积会造成血液在腹部器官（肝和脾）及下肢皮下组织中堆积。
4. Damage to the heart valves can produce lesions called vegetations that may break off into the bloodstream as emboli, which can lodge in the small vessels, causing obstruction of the vessels.
   心脏瓣膜损害可能产生赘生物病变，赘生物可能脱落成为栓子，栓子可能停滞在小血管内，导致血管阻塞。
5. A blood clot may form, causing the dangerous condition called thrombophlebitis, with the possibility of a piece of the clot becoming loosened and floating in the blood as an embolus.
   血凝块形成，导致称为血栓性静脉炎的危险病情。血凝块可能变得松散、脱落而成为栓子悬浮在血液中。

Ⅳ. Discuss the following topics.

1. What are the differences between embolism and thrombosis?
   Thrombosis refers to the formation of a blood clot or thrombus in a vessel while embolism refers to occlusion of a vessel by a thrombus or other mass carried in the bloodstream. Therefore, the latter one results from the former one.
2. How can hemorrhage be managed?
   Hemorrhage can be managed in different ways. Capillary bleeding is usually stopped by the normal process of clot formation. Flow from larger vessels can be stopped by appropriate first-aid measures by anyone who happens to be at the scene. In most cases pressure with a clean bandage directly on the wound will stop the bleeding effectively. Immediate appropriate action should be taken for hemorrhage from a cut artery.
3. Say something about a particular disease of the cardiovascular system that you are interested in.
   The answer is open.

Passage Three Risk Factors of Cardiovascular Disease

Exercises

Ⅰ. Read the following statements and decide whether they are true or false. Then write T for true and F for false in the brackets.

1. [F] There is no way to control the risk factors of cardiovascular disease.
2. [F] The damage caused by smoking to the cardiovascular system is permanent.
3. [F] People who do two times 33 minutes of vigorous activity a week are physically inactive.
4. [F] Diabetes is the leading cause of cardiovascular disease worldwide.
5. [T] Heart disease is related to high intake of saturated fats and trans-fatty acids.

6. [F] Raised blood cholesterol decreases the risk of heart disease and stroke.
7. [F] A person whose mother had coronary heart disease before the age of 60 has a lower risk of cardiovascular disease than one whose uncle had coronary heart disease before the age of 51.
8. [T] Other than being a risk factor of CVD in itself, obesity is also closely related to several other risk factors.
9. [F] A man is at a higher risk of getting heart disease than a post-menopausal woman.
10. [F] Cardiovascular disease can usually be attributed to a single risk factor.

Ⅱ. Here is a list of terms from the text. Analyze their meanings using the word building knowledge you have learned. Leave the space empty if the word part does not apply.

Term	Prefix	Combining Form/Root	Suffix	Chinese Translation
1. hypertension	hyper-	tense	-ion	高血压
2. millimeter	milli-	meter		毫米
3. premenopausal	pre-	men/o -pause	-al	绝经期前的
4. disproportionate	dis-	proportion	-ate	不成比例的
5. unsaturated	un-	saturate	-ed	不饱和的
6. reversible	re-	vers/o	-ible	可逆的
7. dyslipidemia	dys-	lipid	-emia	血脂异常

Chapter Eight Blood and Immunity

Section A Medical Terminology

Learn the following combining forms, prefixes and suffixes for the blood and immunity system and write the meanings of the medical terms in the space provided.

Word Part	Meaning	Example Term	Meaning in English and Chinese
bacteri/o	bacterium 细菌	bacteriolysis /ˌbæktɪəriː'ɒlɪsɪs/	breaking down of bacteria 溶菌作用
		bacteriology /bækˌtɪərɪ'ɒlədʒɪ/	study of bacteria 细菌学
-cide	agent that kills 杀……剂	bactericide /bæk'tɪərɪsaɪd/	agent that kills bacteria 杀菌剂
		insecticide /ɪn'sektɪsaɪd/	agent that kills insect 杀虫剂
-cyte	cell 细胞	thrombocyte /'θrɒmbəʊˌsaɪt/	clotting cell 凝血细胞
		hematocyte /'hemətəʊˌsaɪt/ (*hemat/o* blood)	blood cell 血细胞
-cytosis	increase of cell number 细胞增多	leukocytosis /ˌljuːkəʊsaɪ'təʊsɪs/ (*leuk/o* white)	increase of white blood cells 白细胞增多
		lymphocytosis /ˌlɪmfəʊsaɪ'təʊsɪs/	increase of lymph cells 淋巴细胞增多
-emia	abnormal blood condition 血症	anemia /ə'niːmɪə/	lack of blood cells 贫血
		hyperglycemia /ˌhaɪpəglə'siːmɪə/ (*glyc/o* sugar)	excessive amount of sugar in blood 高血糖症
erythr/o	red 红色	erythrocyte /ɪ'rɪθrəʊˌsaɪt/	red blood cell 红细胞
		erythroblast /ɪ'rɪθrəʊˌblæst/	immature red blood cell 成红细胞
granul/o	granule 颗粒	granulocyte /'grænjʊləˌsaɪt/	a white blood cell that has granules in its cytoplasm 粒细胞
		agranulocyte /eɪ'grænjʊləˌsaɪt/	a white blood cell that does not have granules in its cytoplasm 无粒细胞
hemat/o, hem/o	blood 血	hematopathy /ˌhiːmə'tɒpəθɪ/	disease of the blood 血液病
		hematology /ˌhiːmə'tɒlədʒɪ/	study of the blood 血液学
		hemoblast /'hiːməˌblæst/	immature blood cell 成血细胞
		hemolysis /hɪ'mɒlɪsɪs/	breaking down of blood cells 溶血
immun/o	immune 免疫；protection 防护	immunodeficiency /ɪˌmjuːnəʊdɪ'fɪ ʃənsɪ/	inadequate immune function 免疫缺陷
		immunology /ˌɪmjuː'nɒlədʒɪ/	study of the immune system 免疫学
kary/o	nucleus 核	karyolysis /ˌkærɪ'ɒlɪsɪs/	breaking down of nucleus 核溶解
		karyomegaly /'kæriːəˌmegəlɪ/	enlarged nucleus 核过大

Continue

Word Part	Meaning	Example Term	Meaning in English and Chinese
leuk/o	white 白色	leukemia /ljʊ'kiːmɪə/	a blood disease characterized by the overproduction of white blood cells 白血病
		leukocyte /'ljʊkəˌsaɪt/	white blood cell 白细胞
lymph/o	lymph 淋巴	lymphoblast /'lɪmfəˌblɑːst/	immature lymph cell 成淋巴细胞
		lymphoma /lɪm'fəʊmə/	tumor of lymph tissue 淋巴瘤
mega-	large, oversize 巨大	megakaryocyte /ˌmegə'kærɪəʊˌsaɪt/	cell with a large nucleus 巨核细胞
		megabacterium /ˌmegə'bæktɪərɪəm/	large bacterium 巨型细菌
pan-	all 全	pancytopenia /ˌpænsaɪtə'piːnɪə/ (*-penia* deficiency)	deficiency of all blood cells 全血细胞减少
		pancytosis /ˌpænsaɪ'təʊsɪs/	increase in all blood cells 全血细胞增多
-penia	deficiency 减少	leukopenia /ˌljʊkə'piːnɪə/	deficiency of white blood cells 白细胞减少
		erythropenia /ˌɪrɪθrə'piːnɪə/	deficiency of red blood cells 红细胞减少
phag/o	ingest, swallow 吞噬	phagocytosis /ˌfeɪgəʊsaɪ'təʊsɪs/	process in which a cell ingests microorganisms 吞噬作用
		macrophage /'mækrəfeɪdʒ/	large phagocyte 巨噬细胞
-phil	affinity 嗜，亲	basophil /ˌbæsə'fɪl/	a type of white blood cell that is easily stained by basic dyes 嗜碱性粒细胞
		neutrophil /'njuːtrəfɪl/	a type of white blood cell that is easily stained by neutral dyes 中性粒细胞
-rrhagia	bleeding 出血	enterorrhagia /ˌentərəʊ'reɪdʒɪə/	bleeding from the small intestine 肠道出血
		gastrorrhagia /ˌgæstrə'reɪdʒɪə/	bleeding from the stomach 胃出血
tonsill/o	tonsil 扁桃体	tonsillectomy /ˌtɒnsɪ'lektəmɪ/	removal of tonsil 扁桃体切除术
		tonsillitis /ˌtɒnsə'laɪtɪs/	inflammation of tonsil 扁桃体炎
vir/o	virus 病毒	viremia /vaɪ'riːmɪə/	presence of virus in blood 病毒血症
		virology /vaɪ'rɒlədʒɪ/	study of the virus 病毒学

Exercises

Ⅰ. Fill in the following blanks with the terms in the box.

leukocytosis	tonsillectomy
bacteriologist	insecticide
tonsillitis	anemia
hemolysis	virologist
gastrorrhagia	phagocyte

1. Tony went to the clinic complaining of sore throat and the doctor said his tonsils were enlarged and congested. The diagnosis was acute tonsillitis and the doctor suggested tonsillectomy to remove the infected tonsils.
2. A bacteriologist is a scientist who studies bacteria, while a virologist is a specialist in the study of viruses.
3. When there is a bacterial infection, the white blood cells would get above the normal range in the blood as a sign of inflammatory response. This elevated leukocyte count is called leukocytosis.
4. Phagocyte is a type of cell that protects the body by ingesting harmful foreign particles, bacteria, and dead or dying cells.
5. The abnormal breakdown of the body's blood cells is known as hemolysis. The presence of certain diseases can contribute to the development of this condition, which leads to a lack of blood cells, or anemia.
6. The substances to kill insects, insecticides, are widely used in agriculture and medicine.
7. Gastric bleeding, also known as gastrorrhagia, is the entry of blood into the stomach cavity either due to inflammation, infection or rupture of the stomach lining.

Ⅱ. Write the English and Chinese meanings of the following terms.

1. thrombocyte clotting cell 凝血细胞
2. granulocyte cell with granules in its cytoplasm 粒细胞
3. agranulocyte cell without granules in its cytoplasm 无粒细胞
4. phagocyte cell that ingests micro-organisms 吞噬细胞
5. lymphocyte lymph cell 淋巴细胞
6. leukocyte white blood cell 白细胞
7. erythrocyte red blood cell 红细胞
8. hematocyte blood cell 血细胞
9. macrophagocyte large cell that ingests foreign matters 巨噬细胞
10. immunocyte cell that functions in the immune system 免疫细胞

Ⅲ. Match each word part in Column A with its English term in Column B. Write the corresponding letter in the blank provided.

	Column A	Column B
C	1. -cyte	A. ingest, swallow
G	2. hemat/o, hem/o	B. deficiency
D	3. pan-	C. cell
I	4. immun/o	D. all
J	5. -emia	E. large, oversize
E	6. mega-	F. attraction
A	7. phag/o	G. blood
F	8. -phil	H. lymph

H 9. lymph/o I. immune

B 10. -penia J. abnormal blood condition

Section B Reading Passages

Passage One Blood and Immunity

Exercises

Ⅰ. Translate the following terms into Chinese.

1. basophil 嗜碱性粒细胞
2. eosinophil 嗜酸性粒细胞
3. neutrophil 中性粒细胞
4. monocyte 单核细胞
5. platelet 血小板
6. erythrocyte 红细胞
7. lymphocyte 淋巴细胞
8. megakaryocyte 巨核细胞

Ⅱ. Fill in each blank with one proper word or phrase. Change the form of the words if necessary.

oxygen	bacterium	carbon dioxide	iron	antibody
release	circumstance	hemoglobin	resistance	tissue

The main function of the red blood cells is to transport (1) oxygen from the lungs to the (2) tissues. Oxidation of various food substances to supply most of the energy requirements of the body results in (3) carbon dioxide, and red blood cells carry it to the lungs for (4) release and to pick up more oxygen. The substance in the red blood cells that is largely responsible for the ability to carry oxygen and carbon dioxide is (5) hemoglobin, which gives the cells their red color. It is a protein complex comprising many linked amino acids, and occupies almost the entire volume of a red blood cell. Essential to its structure and function is (6) iron.

Immunity refers primarily to the (7) resistance of an individual to reinfection with (8) bacteria, viruses, fungi, or parasites. Under normal (9) circumstances the immune system responds to foreign organisms by the production of (10) antibodies and the stimulation of specialized cells, which destroy the organisms or neutralize their toxic products.

Ⅲ. Translate the following into English.

1. 血浆 plasma
2. 单核细胞 monocyte
3. 红细胞 erythrocyte
4. 淋巴细胞 lymphocyte
5. 白细胞 leukocyte
6. 吞噬作用 phagocytosis
7. 血小板 platelet / thrombocyte
8. 止血 hemostasis
9. 白蛋白 albumin
10. 巨核细胞 megakaryocyte

11.球蛋白	globin, globulin	12.肝素	heparin
13.粒细胞	granulocyte	14.嗜酸性粒细胞	eosinophil
15.嗜碱性粒细胞	basophil	16.中性粒细胞	neutrophil
17.抗原	antigen		

Ⅳ.Discuss the following topics.

1. Give a brief description of blood composition.

   Blood is composed of formed elements and plasma. The formed elements include erythrocytes, leukocytes and platelets, which constitute about 45 percent of the total blood volume. The rest of the blood is plasma, which is a mixture of water (90%), nutrients, electrolytes, enzymes, proteins and many others.

2. What are the functions of erythrocytes?

   The main functions of erythrocytes are to deliver oxygen from the lungs to the tissues, and to carry carbon dioxide from the tissues to the lungs.

3. What are the classifications of leukocytes?

   Leukocytes are classified into two subcategories called granulocytes which consist of neutrophils, eosinophils and basophils; and agranulocytes which consist of lymphocytes and monocytes.

Passage Two Diseases of the Blood and Immunity

Exercises

Ⅰ. Match the types of anemia with their descriptions.

	Column A	Column B
D	1. iron-deficiency anemia	A. characterized by excessive destruction of red blood cells
A	2. hemolytic anemia	B. characterized by failure of the bone marrow to produce stem cells or by failure of stem cells to mature
E	3. pernicious anemia	C. characterized by deficient or abnormal red blood cells
B	4. aplastic anemia	D. the most common form of anemia caused by insufficient iron intake in the diet
C	5. sickle cell anemia	E. an inherited disease in which red blood cells become sickle-shaped and interfere with normal blood flow to the tissues

Ⅱ. Fill in each blank with a correct term in the box. Change the form of the words if necessary.

vaccine	diagnose	secretion	defense
progress	combination	intravenous	infect

HIV is transmitted between humans in blood, semen, and vaginal (1) secretions. There is currently no cure for the disease and no (2) vaccine to prevent its spread. The best (3) defense against AIDS is avoiding sexual contact with (4) infected individuals. (5) Intravenous drug use (injecting drugs into the bloodstream) of any kind should always be avoided. Several antiviral drugs have been developed that slow the (6) progress of the disease in infected individuals. (7) Combinations of these drugs—known informally as cocktails—have proven effective in improving the quality and length of life of AIDS patients, especially those who have been (8) diagnosed in the early stages of the disease.

Ⅲ. Translate the following sentences into Chinese.

1. The most common type of anemia is iron-deficiency anemia caused by a lack of iron, which is required for hemoglobin production.
   贫血最常见类型是铁缺乏所致的缺铁性贫血，铁是血红蛋白生成的必要物质。
2. Allergy is a harmful overreaction by the immune system, in which case a person is more sensitive to a particular antigen than the average individual.
   过敏是免疫系统的一种有害的过度反应，处于过敏状态的患者比一般人对某种抗原更敏感。
3. Immunodeficiency is a deficiency of immune response or a disorder characterized by deficient immune response; classified as antibody (B cell), cellular (T cell), combined deficiency, or phagocytic dysfunction disorders.
   免疫缺陷是一种以免疫反应缺乏或下降为特征的疾病，可分为抗体（B 细胞）缺乏、细胞（T 细胞）缺乏、综合性缺乏，或吞噬细胞功能不良。
4. Acquired immune deficiency syndrome (AIDS) is an epidemic, transmissible retroviral disease due to infection with human immunodeficiency virus (HIV), manifested in severe cases as profound depression of cell-mediated immunity.
   获得性免疫缺陷综合征是由人免疫缺陷病毒感染导致的一种流行性、传染性逆转录病毒性疾病，严重病例表现为细胞介导免疫严重受抑。

Ⅳ. Discuss the following topics.

1. How many kinds of anemia are mentioned in this passage? What is the most common type of anemia?
   The passage mentions six types of anemia, and the most common type is iron-deficiency anemia.
2. What triggers an allergy and what are the common symptoms of allergy?
   Common triggers for allergy include pollen, animal dander, dust, and foods. Responses may include itching, redness or tearing of the eyes, skin rashes, asthma, and sneezing.
3. What are the risk groups that are susceptible to AIDS?
   AIDS affects certain recognized risk groups, including homosexual or bisexual males, intravenous drug abusers, hemophiliacs, people having sexual contacts of individuals with HIV infection, and newborn infants of mothers infected with the HIV virus.

Passage Three Acute Leukemia

Exercises

Ⅰ. Read the following statements and decide whether they are true or false. Then write T for true and F for false in the brackets.

1. [T] In acute leukemia the affected hematopoietic stem cells produce offspring that fail to differentiate and instead continue to proliferate uncontrollably.
2. [F] The loss of normal marrow function causes the common clinical complications of leukemia such as anemia, infection, and inflammation.
3. [T] Large dose, young age and short period of radiation all contribute to a higher risk of acute leukemia.
4. [F] The signs and symptoms of acute leukemia in most patients include anemia, angina, and heart failure.
5. [T] Central nervous system palsies and seizures may be seen in patients with acute myelogenous leukemia at later stage.
6. [F] Generally acute leukemia can be diagnosed by marrow aspiration and biopsy usually from the anterior iliac crest.
7. [T] Patients with aplastic anemia usually have both peripheral pancytopenia and hypoplastic marrow without blasts.
8. [F] After a patient is diagnosed with acute leukemia, marrow transplantation should be performed as soon as possible.

Ⅱ. Here is a list of terms from the text. Analyze their meanings using the word building knowledge you have learned. Leave the space empty if the word part does not apply.

Term	Prefix	Combining Form/Root	Suffix	Chinese Translation
1. leukemogenic		leuk/o gen	-ic	致白血病的
2. monoclonal	mono-	clone	-al	单克隆的
3. hypercellular	hyper-	cellul/o	-ar	细胞过多的
4. mononucleosis	mono-	nucle/o	-sis	单核细胞生成
5. retrovirus	retro-	virus		逆转录酶病毒
6. hematopoietic		hemat/o	-poiesis, -ic	造血细胞的

Chapter Nine Development and Genetics

Section A Medical Terminology

Learn the following combining forms, prefixes and suffixes for development and genetics and write the meanings of the medical terms in the space provided.

Word Part	Meaning	Example Term	Meaning in English and Chinese
con-, com-	with, together 合，一起	congestion /kən'dʒestʃən/	accumulation of blood in a body part 充血
		consolidate /kən'sɒlɪdeɪt/	bring together to form a solid mass 巩固
		commissure /'kɒmɪsjʊə/	binding together 联合，结合
		compression /kəm'preʃən/	pressing together 压缩
de-	off 脱离；removal 去除	decompose /ˌdiːkəm'pəʊz/	break down into parts 分解
		debility /dɪ'bɪlətɪ/	without ability, weakness 虚弱，无力
dis-	not 非；separating 分离	disproportion /ˌdɪsprə'pɔːʃən/	not in proportion 不成比例
		dislocation /ˌdɪsləʊ'keɪʃən/	separation from its location 错位
embry/o	embryo 胚胎	embryotrophy /ˌembrɪ'ɒtrəfɪ/	nourishment of the embryo 胚胎营养
		embryology /ˌembrɪ'ɒlədʒɪ/	study of the embryo 胚胎学
epi-	above 在……上	epidural /ˌepɪ'djʊərəl/	above the dura mater 硬膜外的
		epigastric /ˌepɪ'gæstrɪk/	above the stomach 上腹部的
eu-	normal 正常；good 优	eugenics /juː'dʒenɪks/	a branch of study to improve genetic qualities 优生学
		eupnea /juːp'niːə/	good, normal breathing 呼吸正常
gn/o	knowledge 知识	prognosis /prɒg'nəʊsɪs/	knowledge in advance about the outcome of a disease 预后
		diagnosis /ˌdaɪəg'nəʊsɪs/	complete knowledge of a disease 诊断
heter/o	different 异	heterosexual /ˌhetərə'sekʃʊəl/	sexually attracted to the opposite sex 异性恋
		heterograft /'hetərəgrɑːft/ (*-graft* transplant tissue)	a transplant tissue from another individual or species 异种移植

Continue

Word Part	Meaning	Example Term	Meaning in English and Chinese
hom/o	same 同	homogenous /hə'mɒdʒɪnəs/	having the same origin or nature 同源的，均质的
		homosexual /ˌhɒməʊ'sekʃʊəl/	sexually attracted to the same sex 同性恋
is/o	equal, alike 等，同	isotonic /ˌaɪsəʊ'tɒnɪk/ (*ton/o* pressure, strength)	pertaining to equal pressure 等张的
		isochronal /aɪ'sɒkrənəl/ (*chron/o* time)	equal in time 等时的
mal-	bad 坏	malignant /mə'lɪgnənt/ (*ign/o* fire)	dangerous to health 恶性的
		malnutrition /ˌmælnjuː'trɪʃən/	bad, poor nutrition 营养不良
mis-	wrong 错，误	miscarriage /mɪs'kærɪdʒ/	loss of an embryo or fetus 流产
		misdiagnosis /ˌmɪsdaɪəg'nəʊsɪs/	wrong diagnosis 误诊
mort/o	death 死亡	immortal /ɪ'mɔːtəl/	not subject to death 不死的，不朽的
		postmortal /pəʊst'mɔːtəl/ (*post-* after)	after death 死后的
mut/a	change 变	mutation /mjuː'teɪʃən/	a change in the genetic structure 变异
		immutable /ɪ'mjuːtəbl/	not able to change 不变的
-oid	resembling 像	deltoid /'deltɔɪd/ (*delt/o* delta, Δ)	resembling a triangle 三角状的
		discoid /'dɪskɔɪd/	resembling a disc 碟状的
pseud-, pseudo-	false 假，伪	pseudopod /'sjuːdəpɒd/	false foot 伪足
		pseudacusia /ˌsjuːdə'kjʊzɪə/	false hearing 听幻觉
-some	body 体	chromosome /'krəʊməˌsəm/	colored body in the cell nucleus that carries the genes 染色体
		phagosome /'feɪgəʊˌsəm/	a swallowing body 吞噬体
son/o	sound 音	ultrasonic /ˌʌltrə'sɒnɪk/	sound frequencies beyond human hearing 超声的
		sonogram /'sɒnəgræm/	image produced by sound waves 声波图
-stasis	stopping 停	bacteristasis /bækˌtɪərɪ'steɪsɪs/	stopping of the growth of bacteria 抑菌作用
		hemostasis /ˌhiːmə'steɪsɪs/	stopping of bleeding 止血
syn-, sym-	same 同；together 一起	syndrome /'sɪndrəʊm/ (*-drome* running)	a set of symptoms that run together to indicate some disease 综合征
		synchronize /'sɪŋkrənaɪz/ (*chron/o* time)	happen at the same time 使同步
		symphysis /'sɪmfəsɪs/ (*-physis* growth)	growing together 联合
		symmetry /'sɪmətrɪ/	having the same measurement 对称的
-therapy	treatment 治疗	hydrotherapy /ˌhaɪdrəʊ'θerəpɪ/	treatment with water 水疗
		electrotherapy /ˌɪlektrəʊ'θerəpɪ/	treatment with electricity 电疗

Exercises

Ⅰ. Fill in the following blanks with the terms in the box.

diagnosis	chemotherapy
hemostasis	mutation
malignant	prognosis
ultrasonic	benign

1. Although the surgery was successful, the doctor said his cancer had spread to other areas and he had to undergo chemotherapy, treatment with chemicals.
2. In addition to audible squeaks（尖叫）, mice can also produce ultrasonic noises—squeaks so high that humans cannot hear them.
3. Sudden and severe loss of blood can lead to shock and death. When blood vessels are damaged, hemostasis will take place to stop the bleeding by forming a blood clot to block the ruptured vessel.
4. Many flu vaccines are not effective because the flu viruses are very good at cheating the body's immune system via mutation, and produce many new varieties each year.
5. When you go to a doctor with a problem, he/she listens to what you have to say, runs a few standard tests, and arrives at a conclusion as to what is wrong with you. This process is called diagnosis. The doctor may also inform you whether you will expect a full recovery or the illness will affect you in certain ways. This statement that the doctor makes about the likely outcome of your medical condition is the prognosis.
6. In some tumors, the cells often grow slowly and stay in the same place. These are called benign tumors and are not normally dangerous; in other tumors, however, the cells can invade the surrounding tissue and nearby organs and can cause serious damage. These are called malignant tumors.

Ⅱ. Write the English and Chinese meanings of the following terms.

1. condensation　a process of becoming smaller or denser 凝结，浓缩
2. pseudopregnancy　false pregnancy 假妊娠
3. chemotherapy　using chemicals for treatment 化疗
4. malpractice　bad behavior or practice in a profession 玩忽职守
5. mutagen　an agent that can induce mutation 诱变剂
6. detoxicate　to remove poison 解毒
7. premortal　before death 死前的
8. mishandle　to treat a situation in a wrong way 处理不当
9. embryoid　resembling an embryo 胚胎样的
10. isomorphous　equal in shape 同形的

Ⅲ. Match each word part in Column A with its English term in Column B. Write the corresponding letter in the blank provided.

Column A	Column B
H 1. eu-	A. above

A	2. epi-	B. with, together
F	3. heter/o	C. treatment
B	4. com-, con-	D. body
E	5. is/o	E. equal, alike
I	6. mut/a	F. different
J	7. -oid	G. sound
D	8. -some	H. normal, good
G	9. son/o	I. change
C	10. -therapy	J. resembling

Section B Reading Passages

Passage One Development and Genetics

Exercises

Ⅰ. Translate the following terms into Chinese.

1. ovum 卵
2. fertilization 受精
3. germ cell 生殖细胞
4. oviduct 输卵管
5. ovarium 卵巢
6. uterus 子宫
7. endometrium 子宫内膜
8. chromosome 染色体

Ⅱ. Fill in each blank with one proper word or phrase. Change the form of the words if necessary.

deoxyribonucleic acid		pregnancy	chromosome
embryonic tissue		identical	zygote
ovum	sperm	division	mutation

1. At the time of fertilization, the nuclei of the sperm and egg fuse, restoring the chromosome number of 46 and forming a zygote.
2. Embryonic tissue produces human chorionic gonadotropin (HCG), a hormone that keeps the corpus luteum functional in the ovary to maintain the endometrium.
3. The nucleus of each germ cell contains chromosomes composed of deoxyribonucleic acid on a protein framework.
4. During cell division (mitosis), the chromosomes duplicate themselves, so that new cells thus produced contain the same number and kind of chromosomes as the original (a process usually termed meiosis such that each sperm or ovum receives only one member of each chromosome pair).

5. In Australia, about one in 100 human pregnancies results in twins, which can be identical and dissimilar.
6. A mutation is any change in a chromosome or a gene occurring spontaneously, and is obviously, inheritable.

Ⅲ.Translate the following into English.

1. 子宫	uterus	2. 染色体	chromosome
3. 输卵管	oviduct	4. 脱氧核糖核酸	deoxyribonucleic acid
5. 受精	fertilization	6. 有丝分裂	mitosis
7. 合子	zygote	8. 减数分裂	meiosis
9. 胚胎	embryo	10. 黄体酮	luteum
11. 隐性遗传的	recessive	12. 基因突变	genetic mutation
13. 妊娠	gestation	14. 生殖	reproduction
15. 分娩	parturition	16. 难产	dystocia
17. 核糖核酸	ribonucleic acid	18. 羊膜	amnion

Ⅳ.Discuss the following topics.

1. What is fertilization? At what time can we say the embryo becomes a fetus?
   Fertilization is the process in which an egg and a sperm cell fuse together to form a zygote. An embryo can develop into a fetus in two months' time.
2. What are the differences between the two types of cell division, mitosis and meiosis?
   There are two types of cell division: mitosis and meiosis. During mitosis, the chromosomes duplicate themselves so that new cells contain the same number and kind of chromosomes as the original; while during meiosis, the number of the chromosomes is reduced by half.
3. Suppose you were lecturing before a group of rural health workers on the gender of babies, what information about chromosomes and genes would you prepare to give them?
   The answer is open. However, information such as females have two X chromosomes coming from each parent while males have one X chromosome coming from the mother and one Y chromosome coming from the father should be included. What's more, it is important to make the listeners know that the traditional view that mothers determine the gender of infants is wrong and that the gender determining Y gene comes from the father.

Passage Two Disorders of Pregnancy and Genetic Diseases

Exercises

Ⅰ. Match each term in Column A with its correct description in Column B. Write the corresponding letter in the blank provided.

	Column A	Column B
D	1. preeclampsia	A. an agent that can induce a genetic mutation

H	2. proteinuria	B. an agent that interferes with normal embryonic development
G	3. congenital	C. a natural loss of the products of conception
F	4. euphenics	D. abnormal state of pregnancy characterized by hypertension and fluid retention
J	5. albinism	E. removal of fluid from the amniotic sac
I	6. immunogenetics	F. the heretical（异端的）research to improve human race by reducing the incidence of negative hereditary gene
B	7. teratogen	G. acquired during fetal development
E	8. amniocentesis	H. the presence of excessive protein in the urine
A	9. mutagen	I. the branch of medical research that explores the relationship between the immune system and genetics
C	10. miscarriage	J. a kind of family hereditary disease which often occurs in inbreeding（近亲交配的）people

Ⅱ. Fill in each blank with a correct term in the box. Change the form of the words if necessary.

appearance	resistance	trait	feature	interact
cell	genetics	mechanism	ancestor	variation

Genetics is the branch of biology that deals with heredity, especially the (1) mechanisms of hereditary transmission and the (2) variation of inherited characteristics among similar or related organisms. To put it simply, (3) genetics is the study of genes—what they are and how they work. Genes are units inside a (4) cell that control how living organisms inherit features from their (5) ancestors. For example, children usually look like their parents because they have inherited their parents' genes. Genetics tries to identify which (6) features are inherited, and explain how these features pass from generation to generation.

In genetics, a feature of a living thing is called a (7) trait. Some traits are part of an organism's physical (8) appearance, such as a person's eye color, height or weight. Other sorts of traits are not easily seen and include blood types or (9) resistance to diseases. The way our genes and environment (10) interact to produce a trait can be complicated.

Ⅲ. Translate the following sentences into Chinese.

1. Development of a fertilized egg outside its normal position in the uterine cavity is termed an ectopic pregnancy.
   异位妊娠是指受精卵在正常子宫位置之外发育。
2. A common method of an induced abortion is dilatation and curettage, in which the cervix is dilated and the fetal tissue is removed by suction.
   引产是指有目的地终止妊娠，常用方法是扩张宫颈和刮宫术，就是扩张宫颈，将胎儿组织抽吸出来。

3. Scientists working in the field of immunogenetics are trying to discover the nature of resistance to cancer, which also has a heritable component.
   从事免疫遗传学的科学家正在努力寻找人体内的抗癌奥秘，其中就有遗传因素。
4. Unless routine screening for mutagenic effects is developed, science will be unable to devise euphenic measures for each new disease condition.
   如果不对这些因素造成的后果进行常规监测，科学则无法为每一种新型疾病设计出优化的防治措施。
5. An understanding of the genetic basis would alert persons from families with an incidence of the disease to the possibility of incurring heart conditions and perhaps cause them to alter their diets and life habits accordingly.
   了解这样的基因基础可以提醒有此种家族史的人，警惕心脏病的可能性；同时，提醒他们注意改变饮食和生活习惯。

Ⅳ. Discuss the following topics.

1. What is the difference between abortion and miscarriage? How do they happen?
   An abortion is loss of an embryo or fetus before the 20th week of pregnancy or a weight of 500 grams. When this occurs spontaneously, it is commonly referred to as a miscarriage. The causes include tumors, hormone imbalance, incompetence or weakness of the cervix, immune reactions, and most commonly, fetal abnormalities.
2. How many categories are congenital disorders divided into? What are they?
   Congenital disorders fall into two categories: developmental disorders and hereditary disorders. The former occurs during the development of the fetus and the latter is passed from parents carrying the defective genes to children through the germ cells.
3. As a genetics specialist, give counseling to a young couple who want a child desperately but they are worried because one of the families has a history of genetic diseases.
   The answer is open. However, the couple should be informed about the possible options they can take before pregnancy (genetic screening) and during pregnancy (amniocentesis).

Passage Three Genetic Counseling

Exercises

Ⅰ. Choose the best answer from the choices given according to the passage you have read.

1. A patient's medical history provides clues to the beginnings and progression of symptoms and signs which may be quite useful in diagnosis, such as __C__.
   A. the pattern of progression in the degenerative cardiovascular disorders provides important diagnostic information
   B. history of more than two spontaneous miscarriages may suggest a chromosomal translocation in both parents

C. early death of infants in the pedigree may suggest an inborn error of intermediary metabolism

D. measurement of proteins can demonstrate the most important feature of a condition

2. Parents may worry a lot about their kid's short stature. The details of __C__ may provide the information to determine the correct genetic diagnosis for such a kid.

A. the physical examination

B. the medical history

C. conventional laboratory tests

D. molecular genetic analysis

3. __B__ has contributed a lot in genetic counseling revolution.

A. The chromosomal location of specific genes from pedigree information for the X chromosome

B. The chromosomal location of many more genes by linkage to specific DNA markers established

C. The chromosomal location of specific genes from linkage to specific protein markers for autosomes

D. All cloned and sequenced genes of clinical importance

4. Recurrent miscarriages and unexplained stillbirths may be explained by a lot of possible reasons, one of which is __B__ disorders.

A. nongenetic B. chromosomal

C. Mendelian D. multifactorial

5. With __C__, the birth of a child with associated symptoms may indicate that a set of parents is heterozygous for a rare recessive condition.

A. mental retardation B. multiple anomalies

C. autosomal recessive conditions D. neural tube defects

6. When offering genetic counseling, an expert will not __D__.

A. transfer information about the genetic risks

B. put the risks in perspective

C. provide a summary of the disorder

D. discuss the treatment

7. It may be sensible for an expert to __C__ when he finds the genetic counseling condition is a Mendelian disorder.

A. illustrate the structure and ways of identifying chromosomes

B. use teaching aids such as gene diagrams, sample pedigrees, and other models

C. discuss the basic concepts of single gene inheritance and center on the mode of inheritance involved in the particular family

D. explain heterozygosity to help clarify the autosomal dominant inheritance

Ⅱ. Here is a list of terms from the text. Analyze their meanings using the word building knowledge you have learned. Leave the space empty if the word part does not apply.

Term	Prefix	Combining Form/Root	Suffix	Chinese Translation
1. reproduction	re- pro-	duct	-ion	生殖
2. heterogeneity	heter/o-	gen	-ity	异质性
3. degenerative	de-	gen	-tive	退行性的
4. chromosomal		chrom/o-	-some -al	染色体的
5. autosomal	auto-	some	-al	常染色体的
6. anomaly	a-	nom	-al -y	反常
7. chondrodystrophy	dys-	chondr/o troph	-y	软骨营养不良

全国高等学校教材
供临床、预防、基础、口腔、药学、护理等专业用

医学专业英语 阅读一分册 第2版

☑ 医学专业英语 阅读一分册 教师用书

医学专业英语 阅读二分册 第2版

医学专业英语 阅读二分册 教师用书

医学专业英语 听 说 分 册 第2版

医学专业英语 听 说 分 册 教师用书

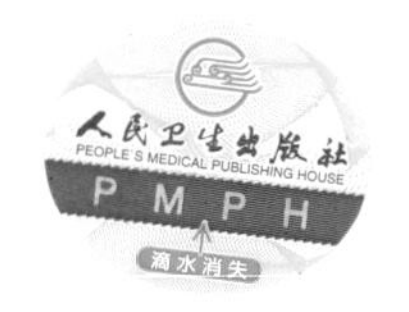

策划编辑 王 暄
责任编辑 王 暄
书籍设计 锋尚设计
姚依帆

人卫智网
www.ipmph.com
医学教育、学术、考试、健康，
购书智慧智能综合服务平台

人卫官网
www.pmph.com
人卫官方资讯发布平台

关注人卫健康
提升健康素养

定 价：30.00 元

国高等学校教材
临床、预防、基础、口腔、药学、护理等专业用

总主编 白永权

MEDICAL ENGLISH

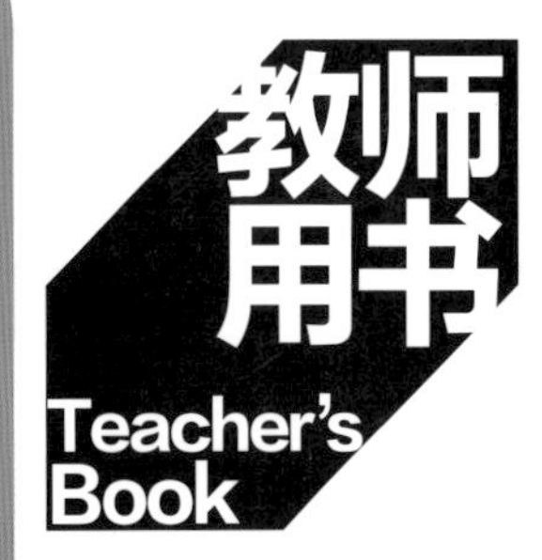

医学专业英语

阅读二分册

主 编 卢凤香

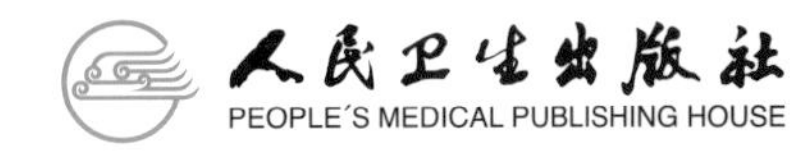